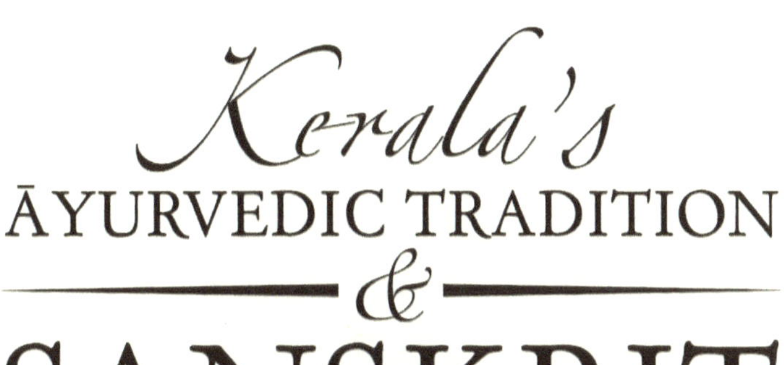

Kerala's
ĀYURVEDIC TRADITION
&
SANSKRIT
SOURCES

AJITHKUMAR K.V.

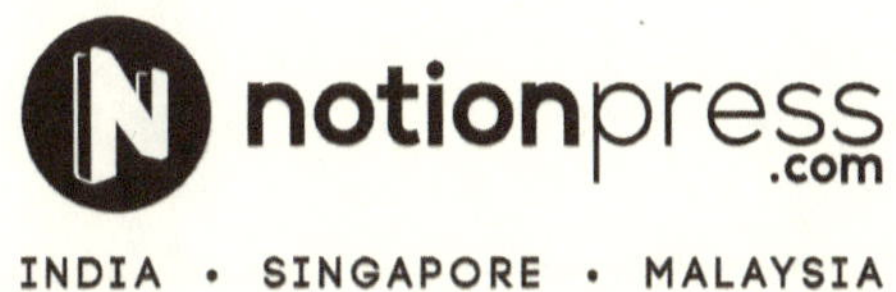

notionpress.com

INDIA · SINGAPORE · MALAYSIA

Notion Press

Old No. 38, New No. 6
McNichols Road, Chetpet
Chennai - 600 031

First Published by Notion Press 2020
Copyright © Ajithkumar K.V. 2020
All Rights Reserved.

ISBN 978-1-64869-993-1

CONTENTS

FOREWORD

Sanskrit language has been a vehicle of scientific thought throughout India and Kerala is no exception to this. In fact, the Intellectual history of Kerala is inextricably linked with Sanskrit as is well attested by the advancement made by Kerala in ancient and medieval times in various disciplines like Āyurveda, mathematics, astronomy, astrology, iconography and Vāstuvidyā, apart from the impressive achievements made in Vedic and classical literature. It in only in recent times that the global academic world has started paying attention to this amazing and rewarding field of Indological research.

As to Āyurveda, as is well known, its tradition belongs to the entire India and has its roots in the hoary tradition of healing stretching towards the Vedic period. Its growth did not, however, get retarded in Kerala unlike in the case of several disciplines of ancient Indian śāstra tradition which tend to show stagnation over the centuries. A close scrutiny of Kerala's Āyurvedic tradition shows a harmonious blend of tradition and innovation. To illustrate, Keralites introduced subtle changes in the whole perception of seasons in Āyurvedic practices, to suit the requirements of the coastal terrain characterized by long spells of monsoon and summer and the absence of severe winter. Another challenging area seems to be finding suitable substitutes for medicinal plants , introduced to the system in the place of its origin, but which are not available in the place of its adoption. In this respect also the great practitioners of Kerala seem to have fared admirably.

It is no wonder Kerala has created a niche for itself in global healthcare scenario through its traditional and time tested medical practices. The continuous and meticulous tradition maintained and preserved in Kerala, like the famous *Pañcakarma* therapy, which are almost extinct in many other parts of India, show the care and devotion with which the physicians of Kerala have preserved India's medical legacy.

From all this it will be evident that vigorous research is necessary to sustain and update our knowledge in Āyurveda, which has emerged as a powerful branch of alternate medicine. The relevance of Āyurveda in grossly neglected areas like rejuvenation therapy and health maintenance is being proven day by day in the present health scenario.

It is a pity that textual and philological studies often take a back seat in contemporary research related to Āyurveda and many treatises of the discipline are not studied or taught properly in the present curricular set up. This deprives prospective medical practitioners some much needed inputs from tradition to broaden their knowledge base and perspectives. Against this backdrop, the present attempt undertaken by Ajithkumar is a good beginning in charting the contours of the textual tradition of Kerala in Āyurveda. Ajithkumar, who worked under my supervision in Calicut University for his doctoral program has earnestly collected information about all the textual sources of Kerala's Āyurvedic heritage in the present work against the backdrop of India's Āyurvedic legacy.Naturally this involves a close look into the origin, development and evolution of Āyurveda down the centuries as a viable health program. Though his focal are is Sanskrit texts, Ajithkumar has discussed the textual tradition in Malayalam also. A cursory look at the history of Kerala's scientific and technological history would indeed reveal that Sanskrit was always interlinked with Malayalam for the propagation and clarification of ideas. Therefore a lot of works were composed in Malayalam also, which have an organic affinity with the texts written in Sanskrit .Of course the seminal works taught and studied in Kerala were written in Sanskrit, among which *Aṣṭāṅgasaṅgraha* and *Aṣṭāṅgahṛdaya* occupied the pride of place, but texts came to be written in both Sanskrit and Malayalam to develop the theoretical and practical base of the science. This pioneer attempt has to be followed by a concerted effort of Sanskritists and specialists in Āyurveda to edit, translate and publish important works of Kerala in Āyurveda.

I hope that this work will rekindle interest among specialists for further research in the field.

— **Dr. C. Rajendran**

Ex Dean, Faculty of languages and Literature

University of Calicut

PREFACE

The contribution of Kerala to Āyurveda is unique. Its popularity in Kerala is so pronounced that there is even a wrong notion among the people that Kerala is the birth place of Āyurveda. This perception is supported by an array of foreigners to Kerala for Āyurvedic treatment.

Even though not the birth place of Āyurveda, Kerala has sustained the Āyurvedic tradition in Sanskrit *Samhitā* texts. It has also evolved special therapeutic techniques out of it. Before the advent of Sanskrit language, Kerala has her own system of healing reflected in ancient Tamil works like *Akanānūru* and *Puranānūru* etc. It deserves special mention here that Kerala got an opportunity to preserve Āyurveda tradition in Samhitā texts because no other tradition like the Unāni was introduced here in a big way. Due to this historical reason and because of rich flaura and fauna Āyurveda flourished in Kerala. Modern physicians like P.S Varrier keep Āyurveda moving forwards by including new findings of Modern science also to this field. Nowadays Kerala is the only place in India where 'holistic Āyurveda' is practised as a healing therapy.

In this background the topic Sanskrit sources of Kerala Āyurvedic tradition is attempted. The aim of the work is to examine the basic Sanskrit text s followed in Kerala so as to study the relationship between *Śāstra* and *Prayoga*.

KALADY   **AJITH KUMAR. K.V.**

ACKNOWLEDGEMENT

I hope that this study would be a humble addition to the knowledge of Āyurveda tradition in Kerala. It is my pleasant duty to thank the several authorities and institutions which helped me to publish this work. Dr. C. Rajendran, Former Head of Department of Sanskrit, Calicut University provided efficient guidance for my work and blessed me with a foreword and persuaded me to publish this work to which I am thankful to him. Dr. Raghavan Thirumulppad, Dr. P.K. Varrier, Dr. C.R. Agnivesh, Dr. N.V.P. Unithiri, Professor of Sanskrit, Calicut University, Dr. K.V. Raghavan, Retired Senior medical officer, Dr. Murali M. Āyurveda, Professor of Āyurveda, Dr. P. Gaurishanker, Āyurveda College, Ollur, Dr. K. Sasidharan former Reader of Āyurveda in Sanskrit University Kalady, Dr. Surendran Nair, Former Principal Government Āyurveda College, Trivandrum, Sri Somasekharan, a traditional scholar in Āyurveda. Sri Thanu.V.G, and Dr. Narayanan Moos, S.N.M Vaidyasala, Dr.Vijayan Nangely have helped me in clearing my doubts during my studies and I am extremely thankful to them for their most valuable suggestions.

I am deeply indebted to Prof. M. Sivakumaraswamy, a veteran scholar and an awardee of president in Sanskrit, Bangalore for his kindness to go through the whole work and made some valuable suggestions.

I offer sincere thanks to Dr. Dharmaraj Adatt, Vice Chancellor and confreres in the Department of Sanskrit Sahitya, Sanskrit University Kalady who have given valuable suggestions and assistance in the preparation of my work.

My thanks are due to team of friends in Notion press for publishing this work. I am grateful to Dr. Puspadas Kuniyil, Dr. Anilkumar, A.R, Dr. K.V.Suresh, my daughters Abhirami, Parvathy and my wife Jeena for their kind support and co-operation in materializing this work. I devote this work to my mother Smt. Radha who always disrupted my sleep during the early hours of day by rising me up for studies and always experienced my fury and anger during childhood days which cultivated the good habit of getting up early in the morning.

KALADY   **AJITH KUMAR. K.V.**

Chapter 1

INTRODUCTION

Āyurveda is one of the oldest living medical systems of the world. It is still being practised widely today because people prefer to have a treatment which is free from side effects. Also there are many ailments like rheumatism which are better treated in Āyurveda. The principles of Modern medicine are ever changing. What was regarded scientific and true a few years back, would be rejected today and whatever is regarded true and scientific today would be rejected in future. So there is always some problem in regard to the acceptance between Āyurveda and modern medicine. The approach of Āyurveda is synthetical based on the subjective findings which are nearest to the law of nature, whereas the approach of modern medicine is analytical based on the objective findings which become farther and farther from the law of nature. Since there are a few basic elements in nature which are by no means changed and the Āyurveda following the law of nature has no possibility of change. Āyurveda, above everything is the accumulated wisdom of a civilization over centuries based on the observation of the working of life and nature.

The World Health Organisation (W.H.O) proclaimed the slogan of 'health for all by 2000'. It declared that the goal would be achieved only with the help of traditional systems of medicine prevalent in the developing and under developed countries as in Asia and Africa along with modern medicine.

Consequent upon this, the physicians and, researchers all over the world have evinced a keen interest in alternate systems like Āyurveda, Homeopathy, Chinese system, Tibetan system, Unāni system, and other Asio-African traditional systems of medicine. It deserves special mention that these systems are nowadays designated as complementary systems instead of alternate systems by modern American scholars.[1] This change in nomenclature suggests a paradigm shift in contemporary thinking which has learned to assimilate traditional wisdom to its fold.

Among these complementary systems of treatment the uniqueness of Āyurveda is brought out by Dr. Rolland J. False (Professor and Chairman, Department of Surgery, Southern Ithinoise University) and Dr. Glen B. Davidson (Chairman, Department of Medical Humanities and Project Co-ordinater, S.I.U) thus:

The systematic approach and inherent features of Āyurveda will have an impact on the medical profession of America. The holistic concept of Āyurveda is of particular significance. Āyurveda can solve many health problems of primary health care in the west. The Southern Ithinoise University (S.I.U) has investigated medical systems in other parts of the world but have found Āyurveda to be the most systematic.[2]

Āyurveda has only one objective to be achieved and that objective is the maintenance of the state of well being or re-establishing the state of well being in the organism. This is also known as a state of equilibrium (*svāsthya*). In Āyurveda, health represents not only the cure of ailments, but also the maintenance of equilibrium and happiness at spiritual, physical and mental levels of the individual. Suśruta in his *samhitā* defines a healthy individual (*svastha*) thus:

> *samadoṣaḥ samāgniśca*
>
> *samadhātumalakriyaḥ*
>
> *prasannātmedriyamanāḥ*
>
> *svastha ityabhidhīyate //* [3]

One who maintains the equilibrium state of *doṣas*, fires and elements, and has regular excretory process and enjoying sensual calmness including that of self and psyche is said to be a healthy individual.

It is remarkable that Suśruta included psychic factor also as one quality required for a healthy individual. The mind-body relation is a recent finding in modern science and later incorporated in the definition of **health**, by World Health Organisation:

Health is a state of complete physical, mental and social well-being and not merely absence of disease and infirmity[4]

Āyurveda believes that an individual is composed of body mind intellect and spirit and also there is a dynamic relationship between individual and nature (*prakṛti*). Therefore Āyurveda regards in the real context of an individual and establishes man's relation with nature.[5] *Pañcabhūta* theory which reduces the material phenomena to the five vital elements of earth, water, fire, air and ether has an outstanding importance in Āyurveda. Because it is like the skeleton of Āyurveda providing support and basis for the entire concepts relating to it. Moreover it provides consistency to the underlying thoughts of each and every concept of Āyurveda. In order to make the *pañcabhūta* principle more practical and applicable practically in regard to biological process of the animal kingdom, ancient teachers of Āyurveda evolved the principle of *tridoṣa*. Whatever physiological and pathological processes occurring in the body are under the influence of *tridoṣas,* i.e., the three bodily humours of *vāta, pitta* and *kapha*. Despite the fact that *tridoṣas* are also *pāñcabhautika*, there is predominance of *vāyu* in *vāta* of *agni* in *pitta* and of *jala* and *pṛthvī* in *kapha*. Seeing the dominant role of *vāyu, agni* and *jala* in life, ancient Āyurvedic seers evolved the *tridoṣa* principle.[6] Equilibrium of the above three humours (*tridoṣas*) is responsible for Health and the vitiated condition of the same causes diseases.[7]

The concept of drug in Āyurveda is slightly different from that in modern medicine. The term drug, derived from the French word *drogue* (a dry herb) is defined as 'any substance or product used to modify or explore physiological systems or pathological states for the benefit of the recipient'. The Āyurvedic equivalent of the drug is *bheṣaja* or *auṣadha* that which overcomes *bheṣam* or *oṣa* diseases or even fear of diseases, and includes any thing, material or means, used for this purpose.[8] Thus even food, fasting, penance, incantations, sleep, sunlight, shade and faith in physicians are prescribed in Āyurvedic therapeutics for recuperation from ill health. There is nothing in the nature (*prakṛti*) which is not a medicine as Caraka observed:

nānauṣadham jagati kiñcit dravyamupalabhyate [9]

There is no element in the universe which cannot be a medicine.

In fact, Āyurvedic physicians prescribe not only medicines, but also a whole course of behavior that would help the recuperation. The principle behind this is the fact that the humours (*doṣa*) which manifest as diseases will be aggravated by things, climate and activities not suitable to the constitution of the body and mind of the individual. Āyurvedic texts mention four kinds of treatment.

1. *mantra*: Incantation
2. *maṇi*: These are certain drugs, stones, beads or those especially prepared forms of hardened mercury which are dynamised by great men.
3. auṣadha: Drug
4. *prabhāva*: Personal influence of the physician. [10]

Āyurveda originated and developed in our own environmental and cultural conditions. The purport of the above can be inferred from the following excerpt in *Dhanvantari* by P. S. Varrier:

In Europe warmth is considered an indicator of happiness, as evident from the use of words warm reception. The climate being cold Europeans feel happy with a little warmth. We, on the other hand, living in a tropical region are fond of cold. If any medicine to generate heat in the body is to be administered to Europeans, it has to be quite strong. Their medicines prepared to suit the body of the Europeans are too hot for us. For those living in tropical countries, an important quality of the medicine is the ability of cooling the system. The medicinal herbs from the Himalayan region are therefore considered by many as more effective than those from the Vindhyas. There is a general impression in India that English medicines give only temporary relief. But the Europeans do not impute the same weakness to their system. It is so because their medicines are effective for their disease but not suitable for the conditions of our body. [11]

The unique feature of Āyurveda is the wholistic and integrated approach to the problem of health and disease and therefore it has more relevance in modern times. Qualifying the treatment (Therapeutics) it lays stress to the fact that it should be such as to cure the disease but should not produce other symptoms, complications or diseases.[12] Āyurveda is not only a science of therapeutics but it advocates more of promotion of health and prevention of diseases than cure.[13] It is actually a philosophy of life which leads to long, happy healthy and prosperous life.

Āyurvedic Tradition of Kerala

Kerala is immensely blessed with rich biological diversity and has a glorious cultural heritage. The flora, fauna and other natural resource systems in the state are a good source of potential raw materials for medicinal purposes. This natural resource base is complemented with an equally rich and diverse cultural heritage and traditional knowledge systems. The medical plant wealth, the strong and time tested traditional medicare systems like Āyurveda and the human resource base are the strengths of Kerala. Kerala is also famous for the bodily culture of *kalarippayattu* the traditional martial art. The Āyurvedic medicare practices in Kerala are unique in the sense that they comprise several special methods of treatment such as the *pañcakarma therapy, massage therapy, dhārā therapy,* etc., not practised elsewhere.

In Kerala, Āyurvedic physicians follow *Aṣṭāṅgahṛdaya* and *Aṣṭāṅgasaṅgraha* which were composed by Vāgbhaṭa who is believed to be a Buddhist. It is also worth mentioning here that there are so many well known physicians in Kerala who belong to lower castes even without the preliminary knowledge of Sanskrit. Thus it can be said that folk medicine (may be orally transmitted) among the lower strata of the society and the martial arts (*kalarippayattu*) among the *kṣatriyas* of Kerala contributed a lot to the synthesis of present Āyurveda in Kerala. In short Kerala has two streams of Āyurveda blended together namely special methods of treatments and preparations before the coming of Āyurvedic *samhitā* texts like those of Caraka, Suśruta and Vāgbhaṭa, etc., and the medicines and methods of treatment mentioned in the above authentic texts. It deserves special mention here that contrary to their counterparts in Northern region, *Aṣṭavaidyas* of Brahmin community in utter disregard to the rules framed in *Manusmṛti,* [14] dared to study *Aṣṭāṅgahṛdaya* of Vāgbhaṭa and other Āyurvedic authentic texts and put them into practice. This represents the latter stream of Āyurveda mentioned above.

The present work is an attempt to trace the Sanskrit sources of Kerala's Āyurvedic tradition in this background.There are some authenticworks in this area by pioneer authors like N.V.Krishnankutty Varrier, etc. A detailed account of the Keralite Sanskrit works mentioned by N.V.Krishnankutty Varrier is attempted here.In addition to the above, the study of *Bheṣajapaddhati,* an Āyurvedic work by a Keralite scholar, Purushothaman namputhiri, is also included in this work.

References

1. N.V.K Varrier, 'Keralīya Āyurvedapāramparyam', *Smaraṇika*, p.122.

2. *Times of India*, 13 February, 1978

3. *Suśrutasamhitā, sūtrasthāna*, XV —45

4. *Physician*, March 1983.

5. Dr. K. Muraleedharan, 'Āyurvedam, aṭisthānatatvaṅṅaḷ', *Āyurvedam Ārogyamārgam*, p.19.

6. *Aṣṭāṅgahṛdaya* — sūtrasthāna, I —7

7. *Ibid.*, I —20

8. *Carakasamhitā*, I —26 —12

9. V.V Sivarajan and Indira Balachandran, *Āyurvedic drugs and their plant sources*, p.6

10. *Ibid.*

11. P.K Varrier, Āyussinte śāstram', *Ārogyamāsika*, p.12

12. *Dhanvantari,* 14 January, 1917.

13. *Ibid.*

14. *Manusmṛti-pūyam cikitsakasyānnam and ambaṣṭhānām tu cikitsanam.*

Chapter 2

ORIGIN, DEVELOPMENT AND FUNDAMENTAL TENETS OF ĀYURVEDA

Like the lower animals using various parts of different plants and herbs as medicines the most primitive of men might have had have some rudimentary system of medicine. It can be assumed that most of the diseases emerged, when primitive men entered into an agricultural civilisation. Due to the high yield of cultivation, food products accumulated and made them inert from doing hard work. A sedentary life style made primitive men succumb to various diseases at that stage.

Āyurveda in Indus Valley Civilization

A clear picture of the growth and development of medicine in ancient India must begin with an examination of available information derived from the archeological remains of Indus valley civilization and from the literary sources of early vedic period. Though the Indus culture reached a high level of urban civilization, its surviving written records are brief and unintelligible and therefore our knowledge of it is deficient in many particulars.

Indus valley civilization has been dated back to 3000 – 1500 B.C.[1] The city of Mohanjo-daro extended over a large area and indicates the existence of an organized system of government. It was well planned and divided into several blocks by intersecting streets which varied from one foot to 34 feet in width. Inside the blocks, there were narrow lanes crowded with houses. Each lane had a public well. The houses were quite spacious, containing wells and bathrooms and provided with covered drains connected with the street drains leading to soak-pits. Every house had a separate bathroom placed at the street side and paved with burnt bricks, which sloped to a corner containing the drain carrying off wastewater. Vertical drain pipes indicate that baths were constructed on the upper story also. The elaborate and planned drainage system is a unique feature of the Indus valley civilization which shows special care for sanitation and health. The sanitation was properly looked after is also evident from the rubbish heap consisting of broken pottery, ashes etc. found in deep franchise outside the city. Trees and plants were also grown in the enclosures. The careful town planning, adequate water supply and efficient drainage system testify to an advanced state of civic authority fully conscious of its responsibility for protecting the health of the inhabitants. [2]

Cultivation of food crops was practiced on an extensive scale. Besides wheat and Barley, Rice, Peas and sesame along with vegetables and fruits were items in the dietary.[3] Cotton was also an important crop grown for internal use as well as for export particularly to Mesopotamia.[4] Standard system of weights and measures was also in practice.[5]

The Indus valley people had close contacts not only with the other parts of the country but also with the west and central Asia. Gold, silver, copper, tin, lead and bronze were known in the Indus civilization. Copper and bronze probably replaced stone as the material for house hold implements.[6] The products of the Indus reached Mesopotamia either by sea or land as a number of typical Indus seals and other objects from the Indus valley have been recovered in Sumer at levels dating between about 2300-2000 B.C.. The finding of these seals suggest that merchants from India actually resided in Mesopotamia. [7]

The history of medicine, being inevitable for maintaining creatures, seems to be as early as the history of humanity. Caraka says: *there is no substance which can not be used as drug ".* [8]

na anauṣadham jagati

kiñcitdravyamupalabhyate //

When these two statements are integrated, it is natural to presume that man applied hygienic measures to protect him from diseases and used drugs in case of aliments right from prehistoric age. Even when he was in the hunting stage under Paleolithic and Neolithic ages, he was well acquainted with his surroundings. He identified and knew the plants, which he used as garments and food. He used stones and other minerals as implement. Animals, which he saw around, were hunted. It is logical to presume that the prehistoric man derived his medicine substance from all these three sources - Plants, Animal and Minerals. This continued ever in later ages when these three are taken as sources of drugs.[9]

In the Indus civilization, there are evidences of tree worship, which indicates great importance attached to plants in human life.[10] On this basis, it may be presumed that plant drugs were commonly used than animal products and minerals as is seen even in later Āyurvedic *Samhitas*. Evidences are also there to show that worship of Lord Śiva and mother Goddess was prevalent in Indus civilization.[11] It may be noted that Lord Śiva is mentioned as the first physician among gods.[12] It means that he proceeds Aśvins, the twin god physician in pro-historic time.

Dr. N. V. Krishnankutty Varrier points out thus:

The Kanmada ball and a collection of Horns of deers, which were escavated from Harappa are the remnants of the medicine at that period.[13]

However we cannot say anything definitely about Indians medical lore, though it may be suggested that as in many other features of Indian life, the Harappan culture contained the seeds of much that was the characteristic of later Indian medicine.

Āyurveda in *Ṛgveda*

A few intimations of a more definite nature are to be found in the earliest literature of India, the *Ṛgveda* which belonged to 1500 B.C.. *Ṛgveda* was the liturgical book of the *hotṛs*, Aryan priests whose principal function was originally to perform sacrifices to the gods, hence the work is essentially a collection of hymns devoted to various divinities. Several of the hymns centered on healing deities, most importantly on Aśvins, the 'physicians of gods'. *Ṛgveda* also contain verses that make passing references to diseases, usually of demonic origin, and to other deities who sometimes were engaged in healing activities. In *Ṛgveda*, Rudra is described as having ambivalent character, who might arbitrarily inflict disease on men.

> *mānastoketanayemāna āyau*
>
> *mānogeṣu māno aśveṣu rīriṣaḥ /*
>
> *vīrātmāno rudrabhāmitovadhīḥ*
>
> *haviṣmantassadamitvā havāmahe //[14]*

Harm us not, Rudra in our seed and progeny, harm us not in the living, nor in cows or steeds, slay not our heros in the fury of thy wrath bringing oblations evermore we call to thee

He is also described as the guardian of healing herbs.

> *yāvobheṣajamarutaśśucīni*
>
> *yāśāntamāvṛṣaṇoyāmayobhū /*
>
> *yānimanuravṛṇītāpitāna*
>
> *stāśamcayoścarudrasyavasmi //[15]*

Of your pure medicines, O potent maruts! those what are wholesomest and health bestowing, Those which our father Manu hath selected, I crave from Rudra for our gain and welfare.

The idea of healing is particularly associated with the twin gods the Aśvins. They were prayed to for healing in several hymns, and some of their miraculous cures are recorded. They were believed to have performed remarkable feats of rejuvenation. They gave bronze leg to a hero who had lost a leg in the battle.

> *caritram hi verivācchedi parṇam*
>
> *ājā khelasya paritakbhyāyām /*
>
> *sadyī jaṅkhyāmāyasrīm viśapalāyai*
>
> *dhane hite sarttave pratyadhattam // [16]*

When in the time of night in Khela's battle, a leg was served like a wild bird's pinion, straight ye gave Viśpala a leg of iron that she might move what time the conflict opened.

They cured blindness, lameness and leprosy.

> *yābhiḥ śacībhirvṛṣaṇāparāvṛjam*
>
> *prāndham śroṇam cakṣasa etave kṛthaḥ /*
>
> *yābhirvartikām grasitāmamuñcatam*
>
> *tābhirūṣu ūtibhiraśvināgatam // [17]*

Mighty once with what powers ye gave *parāvṛj* aid what time ye made the blame and lame to see and walk, wherewith ye set at liberty the swallowed quail-come hither unto us, O Aśvins, with those aids.

Soma, the divine king of plants, is also referred to as a healing diety.[18] An unique hymn in the tenth book is devoted exclusively to the efficiency of healing plants.[19] But the language and subject matter suggest that it is later than the majority of hymns were evolved.

In *Ṛgveda* there is a term *bhiṣaj,* a word which later became more or less synonymous with *vaidya,* still the standard Indian term for a doctor of the traditional type. The *bhiṣaj,* however was definitely a healer of disease generally, for in another hymn he is referred to as conversant with healing herbs. The same verse mentions the *bhiṣaj* as a *vipra,* a term usually applied to members of the emergent priestly class of brāhmins, and verse four refers to his obtaining a horse, cow and a garment as a result of his knowledge of herbal mysteries.[20] It is interesting here to note that the term *bhiṣaj* is identified as a brahman in *Atharvaveda.* [21]

It can be seen that in *Ṛgveda,* there are so many references to the curing of illness by various deities like Indra, Aśvins etc; without giving the ways of treatment.

Āyurveda in *Atharvaveda*

A slightly later text is the *Atharvaveda,* the book of the *Atharvans,* skilled in the performance of various rituals. Much of the materials in this treatise are at least as old as the *Ṛgveda* and combines priestly religious notions with more secular concerns perhaps reflective of mainstream, popular culture. *Atharvaveda* has an older name called *Atharvāṅgirasaḥ*; as the name indicates it contains *Atharvamantras* and *Aṅgiras* mantras, the former used for prevention of disease and the latter used for the destruction of enemies.[22] It is essentially a book of magical charms, spells, incantations for numerous ends, including protection against demons and sorcerers securing the birth of a child, expiating sins, and succeeding in battle trade and even gambling.

Atharvaveda incorporates a large number of charms devoted to the removal of disease so it is the principal source for medicine during the early vedic period Caraka also agrees with this view. *Caraka samhitā* observes thus:

tatra cet praṣṭāraḥ syuḥ caturṇāmṛksāmayajuratharvavedānām

kam vedamupadiśanti āyurvedavidaḥ....tatra bhiṣajā pṛṣṭenaivam

caturṇāmṛk sāmayajuratharvaṇām ātmano atharvavede bhaktirādeśya.[23]

Suśrutasamhitā observes thus:

iha khalvāyurvedo nāma yadupāṅgamatharvavedasya

anutpādhyaiva prajāḥ ślokaśatasahasram adhyāya sahasram

cakṛtavān svayambhūḥ /[24]

Kāśyapasamhitā also observes thus:

Āyurvedaḥ katham cotpannaḥ atharvavedopaniṣatsu prāgutpannaḥ[25]

In *Atharvaveda* disease was believed to be largely due to the vitiation of punishing Gods or to the evil work of demons. The moral god of Vedic period, Varuṇa punished those who transgressed his commands with disease especially dropsy. [26]

During this period it was generally believed that the illness could be expelled by the utterance of the right formulae by qualified practitioners often aided by the administration of herbal remedies and other treatments.

Atharvaveda also contains ideas representative of the later medicine of classical Āyurveda rather than the medicine of the early vedic age.

yadāntreṣu gavinyoryad

vastāvadhi samśritam /

eva te mūtram mucyatām

bahirbalīti sarvakam //[27]

That which has been blocked in the bowels, in the two *gavinis* (uraters?) (and) in the bladder — thus may your urine be released entirely, (sounding like) *bal* .

The difference between the treatment in *Ṛgveda* and *Atharvaveda* is that the former gives more emphasis to magic spells but the latter to medicines. Textual evidence indicates that vedic medicine like that of contemporary societies, was fundamentally a system of healing based on magic.

It is also interesting here to note that the term 'Āyurveda' does not occur at all any of the Vedic Literature. Perhaps the commentary of *Aṣṭādhyāyī* of Pāṇini is the oldest work where this word has been cited twice thus -

kratūkthādi sūtrāntāṭṭhak / and kathādibhyaṣṭhak /[28]

Āyurveda in Later Vedic Period

Brāhmaṇas

In *Śatapathabrāhmaṇa* there is a famous legend of Cyavana who had prepared Cyavanaprāśa. [29] The word *śleṣman* for *kapha* is first found in this text [30] which made an important landmark in the evolution of *tridoṣa* theory. Besides, there are many important references about anatomy, physiology and drugs.

In *Aiterayabrāhmaṇa*, the sense organs and their functions are defined.[31] Añjana (collyrium) promotes the eyesight- *tejo vā etadakṣṇyoryadañjanam*.[32] Presentation and position of foetus is also indicated. Hariścandra, the king of Ikṣvāku clan, who fell victim of u*dararoga* by the wrath of Varuṇa is, mentioned.[33]

In *Jaiminīyabrāhmaṇa*, the legend of Apāla and the treatment of her disease are discussed in detail.[34] Kaśītisubhadra was attacked by consumption and recovered after offering prayer to Vāta.[35] There are also reference of *mūtragraha, arbuda, bādhirya, udaravikāra* here.[36]

Āyurveda in Āraṇyakas

Aitareya Āraṇyaka – In *Aitareya Āraṇyaka* sage Bhāradvāja is mentioned as the most revered one among the seers and having the longest span of life. (*dīrghajīvitatamaḥ*) and as such those desiring these qualities praise him.[37] The five *mahābhūtas* are the basic components of creatures.[38] It also mentions 360 bones.[39] Signs and dreams for casting death are also described.[40]

Āyurveda in Upaniṣads

Upaniṣads contain the philosophical vision of ancient seers, which includes many facts and concepts related to medicine.

Chāndogyopaniṣad - It mentions five types of *vāyu* which have been said as *brahmapuruṣa* and *dvārapa* of heaven and world.[41] Digestion and metabolism have been explained with details.[42] *Nadis* attached to heart are of four colours —white, blue, yellow and red.[43] There is reference about foetus covered by 'elba' (membrane) and lying in for nine or ten months and then delivered.[44] It is interesting here to note that life in plants has been demonstrated here.[45]

Bṛhadāraṇyakopaniṣad — It also contains a lot of medical materials. Different parts of horse are enumerated.[46] Five types of *vāyu* are mentioned.[47] Organs of senses and actions and also the parts of eye have been described.[48] Different stages of dream are defined with their essential characters.[49] Reproduction along with contraception has been described elaborately. [50]

Garbhopaniṣad — It deals with embryology and contains information about development of foetus, congenital deformities etc.

Āyurveda in Sūtra Literature

It also contains a lot of medical materials. *Śrautasūtras* name a number of plants prescribed for specific purposes in sacrifices. After sacrificing the animals, they enumerate each organ in a systematic manner. They throw light on the knowledge of anatomy at that time.[51] In *Bauddhāyanaśrautasūtra* there is also a reference to the removal of the foetus.[52]

Gṛhyasūtras have detailed description of the rites of *Gṛhastha* such as *Vivāha, Garbhādhāna* etc. *Śāṅkhāyanagṛhyasūtra* prescribes pasting of labour room with some herbs to destroy the *Rakṣas.*[53] *Kauṣītakagṛhyasūtra* prescribes *Karṇavedha* (piercing of ears).[54] *Bauddhāyanagṛhyasūtra* has mentioned treatment of baby attacked by fever, *Grahas* or *Bhūtas.*[55] *Āśvalāyanagṛhyasūtra* mentions *Dhanvantarīyajña.*[56] *Kauṣītakasūtra* presents a rich material regarding *Ātharvaṇic* tradition of medicine.

Dharmasūtras:- It prescribes rules for conduct of individuals and society and also cleanliness which go a long way in prevention of diseases. Medicine was regarded as an effective instrument of social life. But it deserves special mention here to observe that from *Āpastambasūtra* to *Viṣṇudharmasūtra* there had been legal contempt for doctors which is discussed in the following section.

Development of Āyurveda from Magico-religious to Empirico-rational

Perhaps legal contempt for physicians begun from Ṛgvedic times itself. Firstly this may be because of the necessity of the physicians for contact with every type of human beings irrespective of their caste and creed. Sometimes the diagnosis needs the examination of pus and excretory materials (Autopsy) of patients.

Secondly the treatment is against the 'Karma Theory' prevailed during that time. The yājñikas might have thought that they would lose their predominance in the society if diseases and impotency are cured by physicians. Thirdly this may be due to the attitude of the society towards physical work rather than intellectual activities. From *Āpastambasūtra* up to *Viṣṇudharmasūtra* one can trace this legal contempt.

Legal contempt for doctors reflected in various *Smṛti* texts can be illustrated as follows:

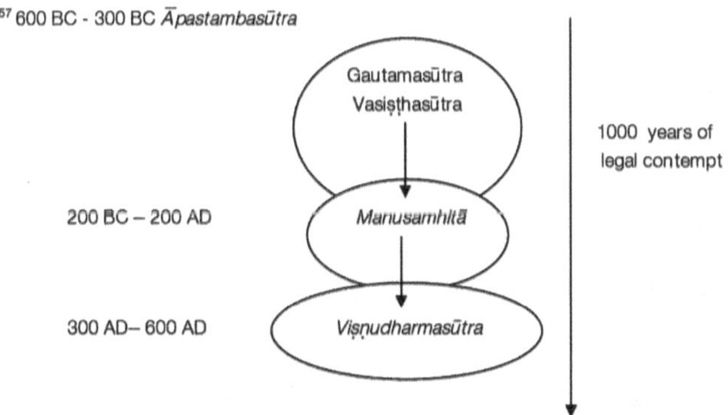

The time span between the law codes of *Āpastamba* and *Viṣṇu* is roughly 1000 years and hence legal contempt for 1000 years.

It is interesting here to note that in one place *Viṣṇusamhitā* takes somewhat realistic attitude.

A *snātaka* must not live in a kingdom in which there are no physicians.[58]

The literary tradition of the *Atharvaveda*, which preserves the knowledge of healing and consider the source of Āyurveda by Caraka and Suśruta, indicates that healing and physicians were outside the general purview of the sacrificial cults. In a hymn of *Ṛgveda* they appear in the middle of a three-fold list of skilled professionals that included carpenters (*takṣan*) healers (*bhiṣaj*) and priests.[59]

nānānamvaunodhiyovivratānijanānām

takṣāriṣṭamrutambhiṣagbrahmāsu-

nvantamicchatīndrāyendroparisrava

Like the uneducated carpenters, Healers repaired what was injured or broken and like learned priests they command esoteric knowledge.

Moreover, their skill in specialised healing rituals and knowledge of potent healing charms and incantations made them comparable to the ritualists and priests of the sacrificial cults.[60] Physicians were a particular group of professionals who combined the craftsmanship of the wood wright with the intellection of the priest. They were respected but were never granted a seat among the ritualists of the sacrificial cults. Debiprasad Chatopadhyaya in his *Science and society in Ancient India* opines that in the early vedic ie., Ṛgvedic period the physicians were highly esteemed.[61] Dr. Kenneth Zysk refutes this view. In his *Ascetism and Healing in Ancient India* Kenneth Zysk observes thus:

Because their mythological counter parts, the aśvin twins, physicians to the gods, were praised in the *Ṛgvedic* hymns for the healing acts they performed, Debiprasad Chatopadhyaya wrongly concluded that physicians in the early vedic period were highly esteemed -an error resulting from his sole reliance on mythological reference in the *Ṛgveda* rather than a more comprehensive picture derived from both the *Ṛgveda* and the *Atharvaveda*.[62]

A passage from the *Taittirīyasamhitā* provides striking evidence to the priestly contempt for physicians, here exemplified by the mythical aśvins.

"The head of the sacrifice was cut off, the gods spoke to the aśvins. You two are indeed physicians (therefore) replace this head of the sacrifice". "The two replied, let us choose a choice (boon) let now a ladleful (of soma) for those two, there up on, verify, the two replaced the head of the sacrifice (hence) when the aśvin portion is drawn (it is) for the restoration of the sacrifice. The gods spoke to those two" those two physicians, who roam with humans (are) very impure". Therefore medicine is not to be practiced by a Brahmin, for he, who is a physician (*bhiṣaj*) (is) impure, unfit for the sacrifice. Having purified those two with the *bahiṣpavamāna* (*stotra*) [63] (the gods) drew this Aśvin portion for them. Therefore when the *bahiṣpavamāna* has been chanted, the Aśvin portion is drawn. On account of that, the one who knows this should reverently perform the *bahiṣpavamāna*, verily the means of the purification is the *bahiṣpavamāna*; indeed he purifies himself. (The gods) deposited the healing (powers) of those two in three places a third in fire, a third in the waters and a third in the Brahmin caste. Therefore having placed the water level to one side sat down to the right of a Brahmin, one should practice medicine. To be sure, as much medicine as he practices by this means, his work is accomplished. [64]

Careful separation and examination of the mythical and human strands in this passage offer insight into the basis for *brāhmaṇic* attitudes toward healers and their cult. *Śatapathabrāhmaṇa* also confirms that physicians (Aśvins) were impure because of their roaming among and constant contact to the humans in the course of performing cures. [65] This attitude persisted in India and is found in the later law books that repeat passages from the law of Manu, stating that physicians must be avoided at sacrifices and that food given by physicians is, as it were pus (*pūya*) and blood (*śoṇita*) and is nod to be consumed.

>*pūyam cikitsakasyānnam*
>
>*pumścalyātvanna mindriyam /*
>
>*viṣṭhā vārdhūṣikasyānnam*
>
>*śastravikrayiṇī malam //* [66]

The food given by a physician, unchaste woman, usurer and one who engaged in weapon business, are considered to be pus, sexual organ, and feces respectively.

Though the law givers are aware of the utilitarian value of the medical activities as indicated by *Viṣṇusmṛti* that it is dangerous to live in a country where there is no physician thoir contempt for the profession is not minimized just as in the case of other manual works like those of the blacksmith, tanner, worker man etc with whom the doctors are bracketed. According to Manu the practice of medicine is confined to the particular degraded lower caste people called *ambaṣṭhas*- those born of *brahmin* males and *vaiśya* women.

>*sūtānām aśvasārathyam*
>
>*ambaṣṭhānām tu cikitsanam /* [67]

Horse rearing is allotted to *sūta*'s and healing is allotted to *ambaṣṭhas*.

Shunning of physicians and excluding them from the *brāhmaṇic* social structure and religious activities imply that they existed outside the main stream of the society, probably organized into sects and roamed the country side, as indicated by the phrase 'roaming physicians' (*caraṇa vaidya*) the title of the lost recession of the *Atharvaveda*. [68] They earned their livelihood by administering cures and increased their knowledge by keen observation and by exchanging medical data with other healers whom they encountered along the way, for the Āyurvedic medical tradition strongly encouraged discussions and debates with other physicians. [69] They were naturally indifferent, If not antagonistic, to *brāhmaṇic* orthodoxy because of their exclusion and their special knowledge was in this late vedic period not yet accepted as part of the orthodox *brāhmaṇic* intellectual tradition.

Several centuries after the beginning of the common era, however, when the medical treatises were becoming established in their present forms, the physicians and their healing art became part of the *brāhmaṇicaly* based Hindu tradition. This is clearly evident from the introductory portion of these works, which recount how medicines was transmitted to humans from the Hindu god Brahmā.[70] The surgical treatise of *Suśrutasamhitā* refers to perhaps an *Epic* or *Purāṇic* version of the myth in which the vedic twin physicians, Aśvins, replaced the head of the sacrificial victim and offers a vedical reinterpretation of the myth as an explanation for counting the branch of major surgery first in the enumeration of the eight fold system of medicine.[71]

Similarly, the medical authors attribute the origin of their science to the textual tradition of the *Atharvaveda*, which, by the time of the final redaction of the medical treatises during the early centuries of the common era, was included with the *Ṛgveda*, *Sāmaveda*, and *Yajurveda (Vedatrayī) in a four fold classification of scared Hindu texts*. This form of authorisation is exemplified in a passage from *Carakasamhitā*.[72] Mention of the *Atharvaveda* here contrasted to the other Vedic *Samhitas*, is significant, for this textual tradition preserved the earliest medical lore. Generally considered to contain material at least as old as the *Ṛgveda*, the *Atharvaveda* was nevertheless held by *Brāhmaṇas* to be a lower order than the other three Vedic texts, a view maintained until quite late. The first inclusion of the *Atharvaveda* in a Indian tradition of sacred *Śruti* texts occurs probably after the beginning of the common era. In the medical literature, however, the *Atharvaveda* is given full authority as an orthodox treatise along side the other scared texts of the priestly order, and its inclusion serves to authenticate the medical tradition in the Indian cultural and religious milieu. These developments signify a radical shift in the evolution of the medical tradition with in the religious traditions of ancient India away from the previous disdainful of the *brāhmaṇas* toward the medical practitioners and their art. The occurrence of this phenomenon may indeed correspond to the fourth or fifth century of the present era, when Buddhism was declining in India and the *brāhmaṇic* religious tradition was making its resurgence through a radical reorientation of Brahmanism. Although considered to be extremely polluting and defiling, medicine was now included among the Hindu sources and came under *brāhmaṇic* religious influences, perhaps out of necessity as the need for the healing and care of the sick and injured cut across the existing sound and religious barriers or, more likely, as a result of the general process of *brāhmaṇic* assimilation.

During the centuries between vedic medicine and the absorption of Indian medicine into *brāhamaṇic* orthodoxy (8th cent B.C. to 1st century A.D.), the medical paradigms dramatically shifted from a magico-religious to an empirico-rational approach of healing. This transition occurred largely because of close associations between medicine and the heterodox ascetic traditions of ancient India. The shunned medical specialists wandering the country side, administering cures to all who required them, and closely studying the world around them while exchanging valuable information with their fellow healers-understandably gravitated toward those sharing a similar alienation and outlook: the orthodox medicants and the heterodox wandering ascetics who had abandoned society to seek liberation from the endless cycle of birth, death and rebirth and who were quite indifferent or even antagonist to the *brāhmaṇic* orthodoxy of class and ritualism based on sacrifice to gods of the Vedic pantheon. [73] The heterodox ascetics, generally known as *śramaṇas*, seem also to have had a penchant for more empirical and rational modes of though. As A.K. Warder suggests that, they attempted to find explanations of the universe and of life by their own efforts and reasoning powers and were particularly interested in the natural science.[74] The physicians began to associate with the *śramaṇas*, among whom medicine developed and flourished, and found Buddhist *śramaṇas* most favorably disposed toward the healing arts. The exact date of the *śramaṇic* sects is uncertain but they were common from the sixth century B.C. Buddhists, Jainas and Ājīvikas were all known to be *śramaṇas*,[75] hence it can be concluded that after the humble beginning of medicine in the vedic period, with the contribution of Heterodox Ascetics and alienated orthodox sects it is developed into a full science.

Branches of Āyurveda

Āyurveda has eight specialised branches. They are (1) *kāyacikitsā* or internal medicine (2) *śālākya* or treatment of the diseases of the organs in the head and neck (3) *śālyāpahartṛka* or extraction of foreign bodies through surgery etc. (4) *viṣagaravairodhikapraśamana* or management of conditions caused by natural and artificial poisons (5) *bhūtavidyā* or the treatment of the psychic diseases caused by the demoniac seizures. (6) *kaumārabhṛtya* or the management of the child (7) *rasāyanacikitsā* or the administration of elixirs for the maintain of youth and prevention of old age (8) *vājīkaraṇa* or the administration of aphrodisiacs.

Caraka in his *Samhitā* observes thus:

tasyāyurvedasyaṅgānyaṣṭau tadyathā-kāyacikitsā,

śālākyam, śalyāpahartṛkam, viṣagaravairodhikapraśamanam

bhūtavidyā, kaumārabhṛtyakam rasāyanam and vājīkaraṇamiti / [76]

It is interesting here to note that the *dīghanikāya* of *Suttapiṭaka* mentioned almost every branch of Āyurveda by name. They are 1) *vassakama* or *vṛsa* or *vājīkaraṇa* (2) *salakīya* or *śālākyatantra* (3) *sallakattīya* or *śalyatantra* (4) *dāraka-tikicchā* or *bālacikitsā* and (5) *mūlabheṣajjānam anuppadānam oṣadhīnampatimokkho* or *kāyacikitsā* including Pharmaceutics. Physicians of *bhūtavijjā* or *bhūtavidyā* and *viṣavijjā* or *viṣavidyā* are explicitly mentioned and both the nomenclatures occur in a separate context.[77] The only branch that remains to be dealt with is Geriatrics or *rasāyana*. It is also remarkable to note that the term 'Āyurveda' does not occur at all in Buddhist Literature belonging to *tripiṭaka*.

Principles of Āyurveda

In India the science of medicine became known as Āyurveda; "the science of living". The term is significant from the semantic point of view, since its first component (*āyuḥ*) implies that the ancient doctor was concerned not only with curing diseases but also with promoting positive health and longevity, while the second (*veda*) has religious overtones, being the term used for the most sacred texts of Indians. The word *āyus* is derived from the root *in* meaning progressive movement and the word *veda* is derived from the root *vid* meaning to know, to be, to think and to attain. Out of these four meanings, the meaning 'to know' enjoys a priority from tradition, while other meanings also have relevance.[78] Suśruta in his *Suśrutasamhitā* derived the term as follows:

āyurasmin vidyate, anena vā āyurvindati ityāyurvedaḥ [79]

Both Caraka and Suśruta concisely state the purpose of their works in their *samhitas* — 'To cure the disease of the sick, to protect the healthy, to prolong life.[80] Thus Indian medicine was a system of so managing the whole life as to prolong it, and to preserve health and vitality as far as possible.

Definition of āyus

(A) *āyus* is the outcome of the combination of a few components (*samyogapuruṣa*, *rāśipuruṣa*). According to different view points, the factors combining together are-

Two — body and soul

Three — body, soul, mind and senses.

Six — five protoelements (*mahābhūta*) and spirit

Twenty four — Mind, Ten *indriyas*, Five proto-elements and eight factors of *prakṛti*.

Twenty Five — Twenty four products of *prakṛti* (inclusive) plus *puruṣa* of which the former are insentient and the latter is conscious. [81]

(B) It is again defined as incessant flow of *cetana* (consciousness) in a particular frame for a specified period of time. Birth, growth, decline, death, respiration, thinking, winking and feeling etc are its manifestations.[82]

(C) It is denoted by specific characters expressed in its synonyms viz. *jīvitam* (living), *dhāri* (sustaining, preventing or the opposing necrosis tissuedeath); *nityaga* ie., always in flux, incessantly moving further, or constantly changing.[83]

Siddhānta (Doctrine)

It is defined as a Law or Doctrine accepted as an established fact after it has been examined by experts in all its aspects experimentally and scrutinised logically and critically. They have been divided into four types as under:

(a) *sarva-tantra siddhānta* — The doctrine upheld by all the branches of science or systems of philosophy.

(b) *prati tantra siddhānta* — The doctrine accepted in a particular school of thought.

(c) *Adhikaraṇa siddhānta* — The doctrine accepted as valid during discussion of a particular topic.

(d) *abhyupagama siddhānta* — Principle proposed and supported with due arguments by a party only for the sake of discussion.[84]

The basic concepts of Āyurveda fall under the first three types.

Theory of causation

Every substance in the world is *kāryadravya* ie an effect or a product. Every effect or product has constituents as its causes, union of which produces the effect. Out of the three sections of Āyurveda, the first section relates to the causes (*hetu*) and the other two sections (*liṅga* and *auṣadha*) are related to the effects. *āyus* itself and even the whole universe are products and their constituents viz. five basic elements being their causes. Similarly, two states of *āyus* 'ease' and 'disease' are also dependent on their respective causes. Knowledge of six categories *(sāmānyādi ṣaṭ padārthas)* is the cause and eradication of disease and preservation of balance in the body elements and health are its effect.[85]

Theory of Creation

Different views about creation of man and universe are advanced:-

a. Successive outcome of grosser elements from universal consciousness, evolution starting from *ākāśa* and ending at *pṛthvī* — these are basic elements that produce by mutual combination the man and innumerable substance in the universe. Their combination in different proportions is the cause for variations of the infinite. [86]

b. Successive outcome of twenty-four elements from *avyakta* or *prakṛti* which is inert and in which exist *triguṇas* of opposite qualities in equipoise and *nirguṇapuruṣa* who is conscious but not active. The *prakṛti* after being agitated due to influence and contact of *puruṣa* gets disturbed in its balance of three *guṇas* starts to evolve and procreate the rest of the elements in succession. This concept of twenty five elements must have been developed by Sāṅkhya philosophy and adopted by Suśruta with slight modification, or vice verse. Caraka instead of advocating *prakṛti* and *puruṣa* as two separate elements has proposed the concept of *triguṇapuruṣa* as a starting point in the genesis. The whole creation, animate and inanimate including human beings is the product of these basic elements.[87]

c. Six elements existing independently combine together to create the universe as well as man. They are the five inert elements viz. *ākāśa, vāyu, agni, ap* and *pṛthvī* plus the sixth conscious element *ātman*. In animate group the *ātman* becomes manifest, while in inanimate group it remains unmanifest. The reason for this difference according to Caraka is that the *indriyas* (senses) are the medium through which consciousness manifests. Inanimate are devoid of senses while animates possess them.[88]

d. Caraka has further clarified that the nine substance or elements namely five *bhūtas* mentioned above and *ātman, manas, dik* and *kāla* are *kāraṇadravyas* (basic constituent) of which all other gross substances in the world-animate or inanimate-are effects or products.[89]

e. Not only the nine substance are causative factors but six categories (*sāmānyādi ṣaṭ padārthas*, viz. *sāmānya, viśeṣa, guṇa, dravya, karma* and *samavāya*) are also causative factors playing important role in all gross products in the world.[90]

f. Suśruta has added a few more subsidiary causative factors viz. *svabhāva* (nature), *īśvara* (god), *kāla* (time), *yadṛcchā* (chance), *niyati* (cosmic order) and *pariṇāma* (transformation).[91]

Pañcabhūta Theory

According to this theory advanced in *Samhitā* texts *pañcabhūtas* are the basic factors of creation. *Ākāśa (ether)* is the first element with only one attribute *śabda, vāyu (air)* the second element has two attributes- *śabda and sparśa, agni (fire)* the third element has three attributes — *śabda, sparśa, rūpa, ap (water)* the fourth element has four attributes — *śabda, sparśa, rūpa* and *rasa, pṛthvī,* the fifth element, has five attributes *śabda, sparśa, rūpa, rasa,* and *gandha*. As the attributes increase in successive elements this process is termed as *uttarottara anupraveśa* or *bhūtānupraveśa* which explains this phenomenon of increasing attributes.[92] This school considers all the five elements or *bhūtas* as evolutes (products or *vikāra*) and hence not being stable or eternal. Only Avyakta and *puruṣa* are eternal in their views. The basic three *guṇas sattva, rajas* and *tamas* of *Avyakta* are transmitted to all the remaining evolutes.[93]

The *bhūtas* are defined as those having specific attributes which can be identified by one of the outer *indriyas* ie., the five senses. All gross products of the world are nothing but the products of the aggregation of the atoms of the five basic elements in different proportions and as such are called *pañcabhautika*. It is the predominance of one or the other *bhūtas* according to which the substance is called as *pārthiva*, *āpya* and so on. This co-existance of all the five *bhūtas* in a product or a substance is called *anyonyānupraveśa* or *pañcīkaraṇa* process.[94]

These are general concepts basic to Āyurveda commonly shared by other systems of philosophy as well. In Āyurveda, there are other concepts which are specific and which have been its original contribution.. They are as follows:

Theory of tridoṣa

The three *doṣas (bodily humours)* are called *vāta*, *pitta* and *kapha*. They are considered as the three pillars on which the edifice of life stands. They are constantly present is the body throughout life from fertilization to death. They are responsible for all activities during health and all disturbances during disease. They are also responsible for death. They are products of *triguṇa* and *pañcamahābhūta*.[95]

So they bear the properties of these *guṇas* and *bhūtas* which come under twenty general *guṇas*.[96] Though they are gross products (*kāryadravyas*) of quite distinct and opposite attributes, they are, in normal condition, intimately mixed in the *bhūtas* of the body. In gross from the three *doṣas* are described as *kiṭṭa* or *malas* and are eliminated in the form of flatus, bile and mucus respectively. In the subtle form they are called *prasāda-dhātus* and pervade through the body and perform specific functions-movements of all types viz. respiratory, circulatory, nerve impulse and muscle contraction etc. Conversion or digestion, metabolism, stamina, reproductivity are the functions of *vāta*, *pitta* and *kapha* respectively.[97]

In pathological condition, *vāta*, *pitta* and *kapha* affect the body by excess of their specific activities and produce characteristic symptoms — pain, inflammation and suppuration (Viscid sticky discharge) respectively. Loss of functions or convulsive movements; rise of temperature, burning sensations and flushes, and loss of appetite, languidity and inertia etc are also respectively indicative of aggravated *vāta*, *pitta* and *kapha*.[98] Thus they are called *dhātus* when they are within their physiological limits; *doṣas* when they produce pathological changes in the tissues and *malas* when they pollute or defile the tissues and are rejected out as excretions.

It is conceived that their existence in the body is, as a rule, at all stages of development and degeneration, which is manifest by their characteristic signs and specific functions. They exist in the sperm and egg cell and control foetal development from initial stage to full term stage. They govern all phases of growth, maintenance and decay. They are the factors responsible for the typical constitution and temperament endowed to the person and also responsible for malformations and developmental abnormalities. They function in harmony and mutual co-operation during health and are disturbed by unwholesome diet or conduct used by the person. Thus the concept of homeostasis (*dhātusāmya*) and dis-equilibrium (*dhātuvaiṣamya*) occupies the pivotal role in Āyurveda.[99] As the moon, the sun and air sustain the universe by their functions of assimilation and motion. In the same way *vāta, pitta* and *kapha* sustain the body.[100] Though *doṣas* are pervasive in nature, they are dominantly located in particular regions of the body, such as *kapha* above cardiac region and *vāta* below umbilicus.[101]

Each of the three *doṣas* is divided into five types having particular functions. The five division of *vāta* are known even from the Vedas.[102] They are *prāṇa, udāna, samāna, apāna* and *vyāna* which are also called as *pañcaprāṇa* because of their vital importance in relation to respiration and other functions. Likewise, Suśruta named the five types of *agni* (*pitta*) as *pācaka, rañjaka, bhrājaka, sādhaka* and *ālocaka*.[103] Vāgbhaṭa, later on, similarly named the five types of kapha as *bodhaka, kledaka, avalambaka, śleṣaka* and *tarpaka*. [104]

The three *doṣas* work under impact of the environmental factors and consequently undergo fluctuations according to change in time (diurnal, noctural and seasonal), age and with relation to food.[105] Similar fluctuation may be observed in three divisions of night. This is more marked and long standing due to seasonal changes. For instance, *vāta* is accumulated, aggravated and normalised in summer, rainy season and autumn respectively. The following table would clarify it.

	Sañcaya	prakopa	praśamana
	(Accumulation)	(Aggravation)	(Normalisation)
Vāta	Summer	Rainy season	Autumn
pitta	Rainy season	Autumn	Early winter
kapha	Early winter	Spring	Summer [106]

The theory of *tridoṣa* forms the basis on which the edifice of Āyurveda is built. All the biological functions are explained on the basis of their role in sustaining life and controlling its activities. *Vāta, pitta*, and *kapha* are mentioned as components of *prāṇa. Tridoṣa* begins and ends with life. They are evolved from the *pañcabhūtas* to take up the functions of life. They do not exist in lifeless things.

Concepts Regarding Digestion and Metabolism

Agni is the factor on which digestion and metabolism depend. It converts the digested substance into assimiliable products and further transforms them into body tissues. Different specific *srotas* (channels) are also there which carry and transport the materials during the process.[107] The *pācaka agni* which is located in *jaṭhara* (abdomen) particularly in the place between *āmāśaya* and *pakvāśaya* known as *jaṭharāgni* is responsible for digestion.[108] The process of digestion and metabolism is controlled and regulated by *doṣas*. Thus *doṣa, dhātu*, and *mala* are mentioned as ground materials of the body in Suśruta's definition (*doṣadhātu. malamūlam hi śarīram*).[109] This definition which is based on the concept can be described as the physiological definition of the body. There are seven *dhātus* in the body such as *rasa* (chyle), *rakta* (blood), *māmsa* (muscle), *medas* (fat), *asthi* (bone), *majja* (marrow) and *śukra* (semen). They are constantly maintained and replenished by the process of metabolism. [110]

Pramāṇas (Sources of Valid knowledge)

Pratyakṣa (direct perception by observation) *anumāna* (logical inferential reasoning) and *āptavākya* (the competent testimony of the *acaryas* of experience) are the accepted *pramāṇas*.[111] *Pratyakṣa* is the perception through observation by the five senses. Any knowledge has to begin with *pratyakṣa*. But there are many subtler things not comprehensible by senses. The testimony of the senses is sometimes deceptive also. Therefore inference has to be accepted. Inference is also based on observation (*pratyakṣa*). Reasoning is the way of inference. The observations and inference of *acāryas* who have sharpened their intellect and senses with discipline *sādhana, tapaḥ* systematically confided their verified knowledge, upto date form, *āptavākya* or Āgama, forming the basis of the study for the aspirant. The Aspirant has to verify the validity of the Āgama (*anumāna* also) by constant application. The *āgamasiddhānta* has to be *pratyakṣa phaladarśana* as Vāgbhaṭa put it.

Idamāgamasiddhatvāt

pratyakṣaphaladarśanāt

mantravat samprayoktavyam

na mīmāmsyam kathañcana.[112]

Since these information described in this text are approved by the ancient scriptures and since its benefits are perceptible these are to be administered like sacred hymns without any discussions (of there efficacy).

Suśruta also says that anything *śruta* (learnt) has to be *dṛṣṭa* (verified) so that all doubts are cleared.

dṛṣṭaśrutābhyām sandehamayapohyācaret kriyām [113]

In short it can be assumed that our forefathers framed Āyurvedic principles on keen observation of natural phenomenon.

References

1.   Piggot. S, *Prehistoric India*, pp. 143 – 44

2.   Basham A.L, *The wonder that was India*, pp. 14-17.

3   *Ibid*, p.18.

4.   Piggot. S, p.155.

5.   *Ibid.,* p.133,

6.   *H.C.I.P,*. pp. 178-79

7.   Basham, p.19

8.   *Carakasamhitā*, sūtrasthāna, 26-11

9.   *Ibid.,* 1.69

10. Basham pp 23-4 & Piggot, p.202

11. Piggot, pp. 201-2

12. *H.C.I.P.* p.181

13. N.V.K. Varrier, *Āyurvedacaritram*, p.26

14. *Rgveda,* 1. 114.8

15. *Ibid.,* 11.33.13

16. *Ibid.,* I. 116.115

17. *Ibid.,* I. 112.8

18. *Ibid.,* VI.74 -2

19. *Ibid.,* .X

20. *Ibid.,*

21. *Atharvaveda,* VIII. 7

22. Dr. N.V.P. Unithiri, 'Atharvaveda', *Saṃskṛta Sāhitya caritram,* p.148

23. *Caraka Samhitā,* sūtrasthāna, 20-21

24. *Suśruta Samhitā,* sūtrasthāna, 30-20

25. *Kāśyapasamhitā,* I.16

26. *Atharvaveda,* 1.3.6

27. *Ibid.,* I.3

28. *Aṣṭādhyāyī,* IV 2.60 & IV 4.102 (com.)

29. *Satapathabrāhmaṇa,* 4.1.5. 1-16

30. *Ibid.,* 13.4.4.6

31. *Aitereyabrāhmaṇa,* 5.22

32. *Ibid.,* 1.3

33. *Ibid.,* 7.15

34. *Jaiminīyabrāhmaṇa,* 1.220-21

35. *vāta evasmai bheṣajamakarot, Ibid.,* 3.266

36. *Ibid.,* 1.254-255

37. *Aitereya Āraṇyaka,* 1.2.2.6

38. *Ibid.,* 2.6.1.25

39. *Ibid.,* 3.2.1.7

40. *Ibid.,* 3.23.10

41. *Chāndogyopaniṣad,* 3.13 1-6

42. *Ibid.,* 6.5.6

43. *Ibid.,* 8.6.1

44. *Ibid.,* 5.9.1

45. *Ibid.,* 6.11. 1-2

46. *Bṛhadāraṇyakopaniṣad,* 1.1.1

47. *Ibid.,* 1.5.3

48. *Ibid.,* 2.4,11 & 2.2.2

49. *Ibid.,* 4.3. 7-11

50. *Ibid.,* 6-4

51. *Kātyāyanaśrautasūtra* 1.3. 32-37, 8.21, *Bauddhāyanasūtra,* 4.8.9

52. *Bauddhāyana,* 14.14

53. *Śāṅkhāyanagṛhyasūtra,* 1.23.1

54. *Kauṣītakagṛhyasūtra,* 1.20. 1.2

55. *Bauddhāyanagṛhyasūtra,* 3.7.27

56. *Āśvalāyanagṛhyasūtra,* 1.3.6, 12.5

57. P.V. Kane, *History of Dharmasūtra,* Vol. 1-2 Poona, 1930.

58. *Viṣṇusamhitā,* XXI. 66

59. *Ṛgveda,* IX . 112.1

60. *Ibid.,* X. 97-6,22.

61. Debiprasad Catotopadhyaya, *Science and Society in Ancient India,* p.235

62. Kenneth Zysk, *Ascetism and Healing in Ancient India,* p.21.

63. *Taittirīyasamhitā,* 3.1.10

64. *Ibid.,* 6.4.9

65. *Satapathabrāhmaṇa,* 4.1.54

66. *Manusmṛti,* IV 220

67. *Ibid.,* X 46.7

68. Debiprasad Chatopadhyaya, *Science & Society in Ancient India,* p.29.

69. *Carakasamhitā,* VI.8.13,20

70. *Ibid, sūtrasthāna,* 1.1-40

71. Kenneth Zysk, *Ascetism & Healing in Ancient India,* p.25

72. *Carakasamhitā,* sūtrasthāna, 20-21

73. Kenneth G. Zysk, *Ascentism & Healing Ancient India,* p.26

74. A.K Warder, *Indian Buddhism,* P.33-35

75. Kenneth G.Zysk, *Ascetism & Healing in Ancient India*, p.27

76. *Carakasamhitā*, sūtrasthāna, 28

77. *Suttapiṭaka,*. Dīghanikāya, I.2-21

78. *Carakasamhitā*, sūtrasthāna, 1.43; 30. 23

79. *Suśrutasamhitā*, sūtrasthāna, 1.15

80. *Carakasamhitā*, VI. 1.4; sūtrasthāna,11

81. *Carakasamhitā*, sūtrasthāna, 1.42, 46

82. *Ibid.*, 30.22

83. *Ibid.*, 1.42

84. *Ibid.*, VI 8.7

85. *Ibid.*, 1.24, 44, 48, 53 & 54

86. *Ibid., śarīrasthāna*, 4.8

87. *Ibid.*, 1.61; *Suśrutasamhitā, śarīrasthāna*,1.3-4

88. *Ibid.*, 5.4; *Ibid* 1.22

89. *Suśrutasamhitā*. Sūtrasthāna, 1.2

90. *Carakasamhitā*, sūtrasthāna, 1.53

91. *Suśrutasamhitā*, Sūtrasthāna, 1.11

92. *Ibid.*, 42-3; *Carakasamhitā*, śarīrasthāna, 1.27-28

93. *Ibid.*, 1.10, 12.20

94. *Ibid.*, 41.3

95. *Ibid.*, 1.57-61

96. *Carakasamhitā*, sūtrasthāna, 26.11

97. *Ibid.*, 1.44

98. *Carakasamhitā*, sūtrasthāna, 20-21

99. *Suśrutasamhitā*, Sūtrasthāna, 21.3

100. *Ibid.*, 21.8

101. *Aṣṭāṅgahṛdaya*, sūtrasthāna, 1.7

102. P.V Sharma, *Medicine in Ancient India*, p.387

103. *Suśrutasamhitā*, Sūtrasthāna, 15.3

104. *Aṣṭāṅgahṛdaya*, sūtrasthāna,12. 15-17

105. *Carakasamhitā, sūtrasthāna*, 6.6-7 & A.H Su, 1.7-8

106. *Aṣṭāṅgahṛdaya,* sūtrasthāna, 12. 15-17

107. *Carakasamhitā,* sūtrasthāna, VI 5

108. *Ibid.,* 28.4

109. *Suśrutasamhitā,* sūtrasthāna, 15,3

110. *Carakasamhitā,* cikitsāsthāna, 15-16-19

111. *Aṣṭāṅgahṛdaya,* sūtrasthāna, 22

112. *Ibid.,* 81

113. K. Raghavan Thirumulppad, *Scientific Heritage of Ancient India,* p.12

Chapter 3

EVOLUTION OF ĀYURVEDA IN KERALA AND SOME UNIQUE THERAPIES OF KERALA

Origin of Kerala

The fact the country called Kerala, stretching form Gokarnam to Cape comerin and lying between the Ghats and the sea was under water is now well admitted.[1] Whether this formation was the result of continuous accumulation of the silt laden streams or whether it was the result of a volcanic action, is a problem still awaiting solution. Legends speak of Kerala as a creation of Paraśurāma, one of the Avatāras of Viṣṇu who gave the land to Brahmins as a gift to atone for his sin of extirpating the *kṣatriyas*. Undoubtedly the story is a later creation to give Brahmins unbounded power and influence in the country.

According to some scholars the name Kerala was derived from the Kannada term *keral* which has the Tamil synonym *cherala*. The word means the land bounded by mountains and seas. But the travelers of the medieval period denoted the place by the name *malai*. Al-Idirisi called the country *manibar* later in the year 1153. The Arabs had in their stock another favourite name, *Biladul phul phul* meaning there by the country of pepper. The travellers Rashid-ud-deen (1247) and Marco polo (1292) name the country 'Malibar' where as Ibu-Batula (1342) calls it 'Malaibar'. Portuguese and Dutch records used the term Malabar to denote Kerala.[2] It seems to be a word gained importance after Sanskrit language got prominence in the society. In Sanskrit the word *kera* means coconut, which is one of the special products of the West coast. Moreover the coastal belt lying between the western Ghats and the Arabian sea in Peninsular India was designated 'Kerala in Sanskrit literature even from very ancient times.

History of Kerala

The early history of Kerala still remains unexplored. What little is known, comes from the ancient Tamil works, the memoirs of foreign travelers, a few inscriptions and from some excavations. The popular tradition is that Kerala was reclaimed by Paraśurāma. This story also seen in other regions of the Konkan coast seems to be a later invention to give legitamacy to the immigrant settlers. Kerala had trade relation with Egypt, Babylon, Phoenicia and is the later years, with the Greecio-Roman world. Moreover the archeological remains excavated from different parts of Kerala prove that these parts of the country were habitation sites as early as Neo-lithic period itself.

Kerala was a part of a larger Tamil Kingdoms up to the formation of a separate state on 1956. The history of Kerala is immersed in the history Tamil Kingdom. The landscape (geographical area) from Tirupati to Kanyakmari was known as *Chenthamizhnādu.*[3] The dynasties of at least four Kindgoms of Tamil Nadu had historical links with Kerala that of Ezhimalai, Chera, Pandya and Ay dynasties. The system of land- division which has been referred to in Tamil Literature, can be said to exist in Kerala also.

According to the oral tradition of old Tamil (*pazhatamizhpāṭṭu*), the ancient geographical land divisions were Kurinji, Mullai, Marutam, Neytal and Palai. These were referred to as the five Tiṇai. Kurinji was associated with the mountains, Mullai with the high grassy plateaus, Marutam with the fertile agricultural plains and Neytal with the coastal areas. Palai referred to the barren and dry lands. The other four land areas could become Palai during the scorching drought. Probably that was why when generally referring to land division the term Palai was omitted and the land of the other four Tiṇais was referred to as *Na-nilai.* [4]

The Tamil land division not only corresponds to the peculiarities of the landscape but also depends up on the social life and the relation between man and nature. The ancient Tamil folk songs (*Eṭṭuttuka, Pattupāṭṭu*) are generally believed to describe the conditions during 3rd BC. to 3rd AD. According to the tradition the people living in the Kurinji. Tiṇai were hunters. They lived by hunting speedy goats, (*varayāṭu*) deer, rabbits and also on the forest resources like roots fruits, honey etc. It should not be assumed that there was no mutual communication between the Tiṇais. It has been recorded that Kurinji residents besides indulging in hunting and the collection of the forest resources, were also involved in agricultural activities. For example the 159th song of *Puranānūru* describes the hunters of Kollimala who cleared the forest and indulged in agriculture.[5]

The Mullai residents were known as Āyar and Edayar. Cattle rearing was their main occupation. They were also involved in shifting cultivation. The songs from 266 to 289 of *Nattiṇai* describes the shifting cultivation of Mullai Tiṇai. Marutam was the land of the agriculturists. Uzhavar and Tozhivar were included in this group. Craftsmen like Taccan and Kollan, artisan like Adiyor and Vinaivalar were also required for this Tiṇai. Neytal was the land of the fisher folk; these people survived by catching fish, by drying sea water and making salt and by also gathering pearls.

The residents of the Palai Tiṇai are Eyinar, Maravar and thieves. This Tiṇai included the infertile and barren lands. Therefore it was the den of snatchers and cattle thieves. Many of the songs of *Akanānūru* and *Puranānūru* hints and also describes in detail the snatching and thieving activities of the Palai Tiṇai.

Each of these Tiṇais can be seen in Kerala also. But they cannot be easily located due to the changes that has come about in the contemporary landscape. For example many of the Kurunji Tiṇai areas have been converted into rubber and tea estates. The same is the case with Mullai Tiṇai. The place name Mullasseri, Mullappally, Mullamangalam suggest Mulla Tiṇai. A large part of Marutam Tiṇai has been converted into coconut groves and dwellings. But remnants of the old connection can be seen in the place names. Marutha, Maruthonkara, Marutholi and Maruthuru are just a few of them. Among the group, it is only the Neytal lands which have remained with out much change. Palai can be seen as a proper noun and common noun in the case of place names.[6]

When tracing the early beginnings of medical science in Kerala, surely the early budding must have been in the Marutam Tiṇai. Because of the fertile and luxurious landscape this landscape would have been the mostly thickly populated. The cultivation in the virgin soil would have increased the produce and since it was impossible to exchange the surplus produce, the ever hard working people would have gradually become lazy and as a result of this they would have become victims of diseases. Since agriculture was mainly dependent upon the rains and the magic spells (worship of nature) were evolved to propitiate the rains. The same would have been used to cure diseases. Since the inhabitant of Marutam Tiṇai was involved in agriculture, he would have had the opportunity to understand the qualities of almost all the plants growing there and would also have observed other creatures like dogs and cats feeding on certain kinds of grass when suffering from stomach-ache or some such illness and world have moved on to the awareness of such a cure. Following the easily natural instincts he would have gradually consumed along with the Mantra, medicines which were mainly extracted from plants. Even today in the villages of Kerala, especially in North Malabar when they suffer from stomach-ache or indigestion there is a custom called *Kotikkumantrikkuka* (fending off evil eyes). Along with tying a sacred thread upon the wrist, by chanting a mantra the person is made to eat pepper and basil leaves. It is to be especially noted that this was done by old women who were employed as agricultural laborers.

In the Kurinji Tiṇai in the course of hunting the fast but non carnivorous animals like goat, deer etc in the forest area, the people were more prone to fractures and bruises and thus gradually developed healing techniques like *Uzhiccil* and *Thirummal* (oil and ordinary massage techniques). Moreover, in the process of bartering the forest resources like honey in the Marutam Tiṇai, they came into contact with the healing techniques there and were able to evolve a wholesome healing systems including their medical practices there as well. Thus evolved a wholesome system which depends on plants and also included massaging. The Massier while massaging must have been drinking buttermilk from the *Kumbil* (a traditional system of drinking form a leaf-woven tumbler) and a few droplets might have fallen or the forehead of the patient and the patient must have dozed off under the soothing effect, absolving him of all pain. It must have been from this serendipity that Kerala must have made its basic contribution to Āyurveda the *dhārācikitsā*.

The main occupation of the Mullai residents was cattle-rearing. While they were grazing their cattle Palai Tiṇai residents must have been in the habit of accosting them and making off with their animals. The Mullai inhabitants, Āyar and the Edayar, must have developed a technique of self defense which later came to be known as *kalari*. The *kalarimarmacikitsā* was a method by which the proponents could inflict maximum torture upon the enemy with minimum attack up on the self.

In brief, due to the continuos give and take among the Tiṇas an original healing system had developed in Kerala even before the coming of the Sanskrit *Samhitas*. The grammar text of the Sangham times, '*Tolkāppiyam*' also points in this direction proves this. Medicine (or Healing) does not fall into six duties stated for Brahmins. *Tolkāppiyam* also refers to *velante veriyāṭṭu*, a system by healing and magic. Moreover there is a reference in the *Maṇipravālam* works about quacks boasting about their healing techniques in thickly crowded places like the market place. There are also references to Āyurvedic medicines among the goods for sale is the markets.[7]

The hunters and the forest-dwellers of the Kurinji Tiṇai, namely Veṭar and Kaṇavar etc might have later evolved into the famous Velan and Pāṇar tribes who contributed much to the Kerala healing system. Similarly the inhabitants of the agricultural lands, Marutam, who were known as Uzhavar and the Thozhuvar might be the later known ezhavar who were famous for their healing techniques. Same is the case with the residents of the Mullai Tiṇai, the Āyar and Edayar who later become famous as the Nairs who were well known for their martial arts and for their skill in healing. It is noteworthy that the Nairs of Kerala were good at Martial arts and *Kalarippayattu*. Thacholi, Matiloor etc were some among the famous Nair families. These people who had chosen Cattle-rearing as their main occupation might have traveled from one place to another with dogs for protection fearing the attacks of the Palai residents. Probably that is why the Āyar and Edayar later came to be known as 'Nair' (*Nāy* - means dog in Malayalam)

Thus it is through the give-and-take that the residents of the Marutam Tiṇai, Mullai Tiṇai, Kurunji Tiṇai formulated the Kerala Vaidya tradition.

Keraliya Āyurveda based on Sanskrit Samhitas

Keraliya Āyurveda based on the Sanskrit *Samhitā* which evolved around the five elements and *tridoṣasiddhānta* might have been introduced along with the Sanskrit language. Among such Sanskrit works introduced at this time and got popularity was the *Aṣṭāṅgahṛdaya* of Vāgbhaṭa. Those who followed this tradition of healing must have come to be known as the *aṣṭavaidyas*. The contribution of the *aṣṭavaidya* to the Āyurveda deserves special mention. The eight fold methods of treatment-*kāyacikitsā* (General medicine), *bālacikitsā* (Pediatrics), *viṣacikitsā* (Toxicology), *grahaciktsā* (Demonology), *ūrdhvāṅgacikitsā* (ENT), *śalyatantra* (Surgery), *rasāyana cikitsā* (Rejuvenation), and *vājīkaraṇacikitsā* (Virilification) were learnt and taught by these brāhmins who were known as the *aṣṭavaidyas*. Among these author of *Ālattiyūrmaṇipravālam* of Ālattiyūrnambi deserves special mention. Curing or Healing was considered to be a low-class job, Autopsy and surgery were ostriacized during this period of *cāturvarṇya*. Therefore these brahmins were not allowed to take part in *yāgas* (sacrifices) though they were Nambūtiri brāhmins. They were known by the name – Mūsad, Nambi etc. It was these families who retained the originality and flavor of *aṣṭavaidya* through the Gurukula system. It deserves special mention to note that Vaidyamathom family' is the only brāhmin vaidya family admitted to yāgaśālas.

The existing system of Āyurveda has been formed taking into account these two streams ie., Sanskrit stream and non Sanskrit streams. The role of latter was attested by N.V.K. Varrier- *Ārogyakalpadruma* was written by Kaikkulaṅgara Rama varrier, who according to M. K. Vaidiar often visited the Ezhava houses to study the manuscripts.[8] In the article titled, 'Kerala's Āyurvedic Tradition' N.V. K.Varrier and P.S Varrier have admitted to following the same procedure while writing books.

In short it can be seen that the Āyurvedic tradition existing in Kerala at present is mainly a composite mixture of tradition which existed before the coming of Sanskrit *Samhitas* and the tradition which was enriched by the *Aṣṭavaidya* tradition of Sanskrit based on *Aṣṭāṅgahṛdaya* and other Sanskrit *Samhitas* like Caraka and Suśruta etc.

Unique therapies of Kerala

There are some unique therapies prevailing in Kerala which cannot be seen in any authentic Āyurvedic text. They are *dhārā* therapy, *uzhiccil, ilakkizhi, nārāññākkizhi, poṭikkizhi, navadhānyakkizhi, nellikkāttaḷam, urovasti* and *pizhiccil.* A brief description of the above therapies is attempted in the following section

Śirodhārā or pouring oil, etc over the head

It is one of the excellent therapies for the treatment of several diseases connected with head, neck, eyes, ears, nose, throat and nervous system. *Dhārākalpa* describes the benefits of dhārā treatment thus:

> *Dhātūnām dṛḍhatām karoti*
>
> *Vṛṣatām dehāgnivarṇaujasām*
>
> *sthairyam pāṭavamindriyasya*
>
> *jaraso māndyam ciram jīvitam /*
>
> *asthnām bhaṅgamapākaroti*
>
> *nitaramdoṣān samīrādikān*
>
> *sarvasnehakṛtā sukheṣṇa*
>
> *subhagā sarvāṅgadhārā nṛṇām //* [9]

Dhārā treatment improves physical strength, sexual potency, good appetite and good colour. It also strengthens the constituent elements of the body, strengthens the bones, removes the old age problems and provides almost good health and longevity to the human beings.

During this therapy, medicated oil, milk or buttermilk is poured on the forehead between the eye-brows in a continues stream. If oil is used, this therapy, then it is called *dugdhadhārā*. If however, buttermilk is used for administering this therapy, then it is called *takradhārā*.[10] (See the illustrations at the end of the work)

Tailadhārā

The patient is made to lie on his back on a wooden table specially prepared for this therapy. First of all, the head of the patient is smeared with medicated oil. Thereafter, the body of the patient is also massaged with this oil. The patient's head is also slightly elevated position preferably over a pillow. After examining the patient appropriate oil is selected by the physician. Generally two attendants are needed for this therapy. One of them should hold the vessel containing the liquid, so that the drip falls exactly on the forehead between the two eye-brows and the other collects the oil from the vessel kept below and puts it again on the oil vessel from where the oil comes in drips.

For keeping the oil, milk or Buttermilk, a vessel is specially prepared. Generally, a wide mouthed earthen basin having a capacity of about 2-5 liters is used for this purpose. The basin should be shallow about 15cm deep, wide-mouthed having a bottom with curvature. It should be smooth, both inside and outside and strong enough to bear the stress and strain of the oil and its handling by the attendants. It can be made of backed-mud, glass, gold, silver, wood, porcelain or stainless steel.[11] Through strings or metallic chains, it should be tied round its brim near the mouth and hanged over the head of the patient from the roof or from a specially designed stand. A small hole is made at the bottom of this basin. Over the hole, a small semi-spherical hollow cup should be placed. Traditionally, a hard shell of coconut is used for this purpose. Over the top of the cup, there should be a hole corresponding to the hole of the basin, so that the oil should fall exactly on the forehead of the patient.

This process continues for about 1.5 hrs. Throughout the therapy, the patient should be down on his back and should not move his body. This therapy is given daily for about seven to fourteen days depending up on the nature and mental conditions of the patient. This therapy is better administered in the early morning and should never be given in the afternoon or night.[12]

Manufacture of Medicated oil

One Kilogram of the root *bala* (*sida rhombifolia*) is added with 16 liters of water, boiled and reduced to 4 liters. The decoction is then filtered out. To this decoction, one liter of sesame oil and 250 grams of the paste of the root *bala* is added. The oil is then cooked over mild fire. When the paste become sticky, one liter of cow's milk is added to it and further boiled till the paste becomes rough to touch when rolled between two fingers. If this paste is placed over the flame, then there will be no cracking noise. The cooking vessel is then removed from the oven and allowed to cool down. Thereafter, the oil is taken out by filtering and squeezing out the paste. This medicated oil is generally used for *tailadhārā* therapy. Traditionally, some physicians use cow's ghee in the place of sesame oil is this preparation for better therapeutic results. If this medicated ghee is used in this therapy then it is called *ghṛtadhārā*.[13]

Dugdhadhārā

If instead of medicated oil milk is used in this therapy, it is called *dugdhadhārā*. This is very useful for persons suffering from insanity, sleeplessness, burning sensation, giddiness and paralysis.

In the place of cow's milk, milk collected from a lady (human breast milk) can also be used in this therapy with considerable advantage.[14] It is specially used in the cases of delirium, sleeplessness, unconsciousness and chronic fever.

The patient after this therapy should be allowed to take rest for an hour before resuming his work.

Takra Dhārā

Two Kilograms of the pulp of *āmalakī* (*Emblica officianalis*) should be boiled by adding eight litres of water till it is reduced to one litre. The decoction is then strained through a cloth and added with one litre of buttermilk. For preparing buttermilk, half a litre of cow's milk should be boiled, added with fermenting material and kept overnight. To this half a litre of water is added and churned till the butter portion of it comes out. The butter is then taken out and only the liquid portion is used in this therapy added with the decoction of *āmalakī*.[15]

Before administering this therapy, the head and body of the patient should be anointed with medicated oil.

Traditionally, one litre of cow's milk is added to four litres of water. To this, 50gms of the crushed tubers of *musta* (*cyperus rotundas*) which is tied in a cloth in the form of a bolus, is added. After boiling the milk is reduced to 1 litre, the pot is then removed from the oven. The bundle of musta-powder is then squeezed to take out all the liquid from it and added to the milk. The same milk is then allowed to cool-down. In to this milk, when it is slightly warm, some sour buttermilk is added and kept overnight. Next morning, the decoction of *āmalakī* (*Emblica officinalis*) is added to it and churned till the fat portion of it comes out. It is then strained through a cloth and used for the therapy. This therapy is given to the patient daily for about 10 minutes.[16]

Benefits

This type of *dhārā* therapy cures the premature graying of the hair, fatigue, instability in gait, headache, giddiness, aching pain and burning sensation in the palms and soles of feet. It is very useful for different types of heart diseases and diseases of the eyes, ears, nose and throat. It promotes digestion and corrects anorexia, vomiting and lack of appetite. [17] It also promotes eye-sight and cures cataract in its early stage. It is an excellent cure for chronic in somania (sleeplessness) and often the patient who had no sleep for years together tends to get sound sleep on the table even while administering the therapy. [18]

Śirovasti (Oleation of Head)

Keeping oil over the head with the help of a tubular leather cap (Sac) is called *Śirovasti*.

After the patient's body is cleansed by the administration of emetic therapy etc, the patient should be given oleation and fomentation therapies. Then, he should be made to sit over a stool having the height up to his knees. Thereafter, the cap specially made for this, should be placed over head. Then, with the help of the belt, it should be made tight. The flour of black gram should be made to paste by adding warm water.

Thus paste should be applied inside cap over the head to prevent leakage of oil over this, the oil medicated by cooking with appropriate drugs should be poured when it is lukewarm. The level of the medicated oil should be up to 2cm above the hair roof.[19] This medicated oil should be kept over the head till the patient exudes oily substances from the face, ears and nose, and till he gets relief from his painful symptoms. [20]

Thereafter, the oil should be taken and of the cap and then the belt, the paste of black gram and the cap should be removed. Thereafter, the head, shoulders, neck and back should be given gentle massage. The patient should then be given bath with lukewarm water. Wholesome diet should then be given to him. This therapy should be repeated daily for three, five or seven days.

Benefits

It cures following ailments such as facial paralysis, sleeplessness, dryness of mouth, dryness of nose, cataract and headache and other head diseases. [21] (See the illustrations at the end of the work)

Uzhiccil (Massage Therapy)

Vāgbhaṭa in his *Aṣṭāṅgahṛdaya* points out the benefit of massage therapy thus:

Abhyaṅgamācaret nityam sa jarāśramavātahā

Dṛṣṭiprasādapuṣṭyāyuḥ svapnasutvaktvadārḍhyakṛt

śiraḥ śravaṇapādeṣu tam viśeṣeṇa śīlayet [22]

A person with a view to preserving and promoting his positive health and preventing and curing his diseases should use massage therapy every day. It has the following specific attributes: It prevents and corrects ageing process (*jarā*), It helps a person to overcome fatigue (*śrama*) because of routine hard work in life. It prevents and corrects disorders caused by the affliction of the nervous system (*vāta),* It promotes eye sight (*dṛṣṭi prasāda*), It helps nourishment (*puṣṭi* of body), It promotes longevity (*āyus*) of an individual, It helps the individual to get sleep (*svapna*) and It promotes sturdiness (*dārḍhya*) of the individual.

Among the other therapies like *netracikitsā, viṣacikitsā* etc, developed in Kerala, massage therapy deserves special mention because now-a-days also this has been practiced by Keralite physicians with some special branches of it which cannot be seen anywhere in other parts of India. Actually massage therapy is evolved out of *pañcakarma* therapy. Generally it is recommended to do before *pañcakarma* and now technically included under *pañcakarma*. But it has also been practiced as an independent treatment especially in Kerala. *Pañcakarma* therapy primarily aims at cleansing the body of its accumulated impurities and nourishing the tissues. Once this is achieved, it becomes very easy to rejuvenate these tissues and prevent the process of ageing. The span of life is thus prolonged and the individual leads a disease free old age. One becomes capable of serving the society with ones accumulated experience without any metal disability and physical decay. Even if one succumbs to a disease, this *pañcakarma* therapy, if administered properly, makes one body more receptive to other remedies and those recipes produce the curing effect even when administered is smaller dose and for less number of days. Massage therapy is advised after *pañcakarma* therapy.

Unfortunately, because of historical reasons like political turmoil this classical form of massage treatment went out of practice else wherein India, and in its place, only decoctions were used both for the prevention and cure of diseases. In Kerala however, Āyurvedic physicians kept this classical tradition alive, and in view of the importance and therapeutic utility both for healthy persons as well as patients, its practice is now being revived in other parts of India and even abroad. It is significant that Kerala could preserve this tradition in its pristine purity whereas in other places, it was superseded by other alien medical systems.

The term *pañcakarma* literally means five *(pañca)* specialized therapies *(karma)*. The therapies which are included under this collective term are as follows.

> *vamanakarma or emetic therapy.*

> *virecanakarma or purgation Therapy*

> *nirūhakarma or a therapy administered through medicated enema containing decoction of drugs, among others.*

> *anusvānakarma or therapy administered through medicated enema containing medicated oils among others.*

> *nasyakarma or inhalation therapy.* [23]

Suśruta's school which deals with surgery includes *rakta-mokṣaṇa karma* or blood letting therapy in the place *nasyakarma* or inhalation therapy. [24]

It is necessary at this state to make it clear that these therapies do not imply simple administration of emesis, purgation, enema or nasal drops as is conventionally understood. Elaborate methods are described for the preparation of therapies, their methods of administration, preparation of the individual prior to the administration of these therapies and the management of the patient (or the healthy person) after the therapy is administered.

Prior to the administration of these therapies, the body of the patient is to be suitably prepared and the therapeutic measures used for this purpose are called *pūrvakarma* or preparatory therapies. These are two in number as follows.

> (a) *snehanakarma or oleation therapy and*

> *svedanakarma or fomentation therapy.*

snehanakarma or oleation therapy is administered in two ways, viz. externally *(bāhyasnehana)* and internally *(ābhyantarasnehana)*. The external form is given through different type of massage with the help of ordinary or medicated oil and power and pastes of medicine plants as well as animal products including chemical preparations using metals. To keep the body healthy and to prevent as well as cure manifested diseases, this massage should be done every day either over the whole body or over different specific parts of the body. During the course of time some special massage therapies have been developed in Āyurveda and are still in practice in Kerala. These special massage therapies cause both oleation and fomentation of the body. Apart from curing some of the obstinate and otherwise incurable diseases, these special massage therapies help in rejuvenating the body. If used periodically, they prevent the ageing process while simultaneously preventing the manifestation of diseases. Thus massage apart from its utility as a preparatory measure for other therapies included under *pañcakarma* is specialised therapy with its own merit .

Kerala has evolved certain massage therapies which are very popular now. They are Navarakkizhi (piṇḍasveda), Ilakkizhi (patrapoṭalasveda)), Nāraṅṅākkizhi (lemonboluse), Poṭikkizhi (cūrṇa boluse), Navadhānyakkizhi (ninegrains boluse), Nellikkāttalam (myrobalan boluse), Urovasti (purgation) and Pizhiccil (Kāyaseka) are some among them which deserve special mention. [25] Generally, these type of therapies are used by healthy person for the purpose of rejuvenation. In addition, to these are also administered to different types of patients for curing of their diseases. (See the illustrations at the end of the work)

Navarakkizhi (piṇḍasveda)

It is one of the most popular therapies used for the purpose of rejuvenation of the body. It is a process by which, the whole body or a part of it is made to perspire by the application of certain medicinal puddings followed by massage. The commonly followed method is given below.

Preparation of Decoction and Pudding

The root of the plant called *bala* (*sida rhombifolia*) is popularly used for this therapy. About 500 gms of the root of this plant is used for this purpose. After being washed properly, cut into chips and crushed well, those roots are put into eight liters of water approximately. This is then boiled till the water evaporates and two liters of it remains. Half of this decoction i.e. approximately one liter is added with 1liter of cow's milk and the other one liter of decoction is kept for use at a later stage. To the above decoction add the milk (one liter each about 500gms of rice) (dehusked paddy) is added and cooked till it becomes semi-solid like a pudding. Generally, this pudding is called *payasam* (milk and rice preparation). A type of paddy called *nivara* or *navara* (Oryzapicta), is generally used for this preparation. This *navara* paddy is again of two types- one is of white colour and other is blackish white. It is the former which is very useful for this therapy. In case of its non- availability, even though it is very cheap, ordinary type of rice may also used by the physician for the preparation of this padding or milk product (*payasam*). It is important also that the rice should be absolutely free from any husk. It is particular have to note that for this recipe, rice collected from raw and unboiled (paddy) is to be used. It is not necessary to wash this rice with water before boiling. After dehusking the paddy, rice should be cleaned. After removing the parts of the husk, stone and other foreign material, it should be added to the mixture of the decoction and the milk for cooking. It is desirable to crush the rice grains into small pieces before boiling. [26]

Cloth pieces

Eight pieces of new clean cloth which are moderately smooth and tough to withstand the strain of the process that will follow, should be taken. Each piece should be 40 cm in length and breadth and its edges should be well stitched so that threads do not come out of its loose ends during the process of application of the therapy.

Preparation of Boluses

Pudding prepared according to the process described above should be divided into eight equal parts and kept in these eight pieces of cloth. The edges of these cloth pieces should be gathered together and tied with the help of a thick thread separately to form eight boluses (bundles). The ends of the cloth pieces should be left free i.e. united to facilitate holding them easily with hand by the masseure during massage. Generally physicians prefer to perform some religious rituals just at the beginning of the therapy. Before massage with the help of these bundles of pudding, the body of the patient should be properly prepared.[27]

Application of Oil

The body of the patient should be anointed with medicated oil. The oil to be applied over the head should be slightly different from the oil to be applied over the body. The oil of the head should not be very greasy, whereas the one of the body is normally very greasy. Different types of medicated oils are used depending up on the purpose for which the therapy is administered. For healthy persons and for the purpose of rejuvenation different types of oils are used.

Procedures

The pudding –bundles should be placed in a pan and put on an oven and allowed to become warm. These bundles during the process of massage, loose heat and become gradually cold. In this therapy it is essential that all through the process a uniform temperature should be maintained, and therefore, the warmth of these pudding-bundles should be continuously uniform. For this purpose these pudding bundles should be repeatedly immersed in the boiling decoction and milk. The oven which is used for boiling the decoction should be free from smoke and excess of heat to prevent irritation and discomfort by the patient and the masseurs. The room should be well-ventilated and well lighted ensuring that that the patient is not exposed to draughts, dust or direct sun rays, to ensure this, the doors, windows of the room should be provided with curtains made of thin fabrics.

Four masseurs are required to apply this therapy. A part from the physician, who will be supervising the process, there should be another attendant who will help in collecting the cold bundles from the masseurs and supplying warm ones to them from the boiling decoction. The masseurs should be quiet and fully attentive to their duty. If a female patient has to be given this therapy, then it is better to employ female masseurs and attendants should maintain absolute decorum during the process of the therapy. The room should be too spacious for free movement of the attendants and the supervising physician. It should be secluded and away from the residential areas to maintain privacy of the patient.[28]

The patient will have to remove his clothes and should wear only a loin cloth or under wear. Four of these eight pudding bundles are to be taken by the four masseurs. Earlier these bundles are kept in mixture of milk and decoction and made tolerably warm. Thereafter, these bundles are to be hold outside for four or five minutes to reduce excessive heat and to make them comfortably warm for the massage. Each masseur should take one of these bundles which should be held by the right hard by its tuft and then the base of the pudding-bundles to be placed over the back of the left hand to check the heat.

Therefore, the masseurs should start giving massage to the patient. The direction of the massage should always from upwards to downwards beginning from the neck area. Two of these masseurs remain in the right side of the patient and the remaining two on the left side. Two of them standing near the head should give massage from neck to the hip and other two standing near the thighs should give massage from the hip to the sole of the foot. On both sides, massage should be given simultaneously and at the same time. Every care should be taken to ensure uniformity of temperature and pressure on all parts of the body.

When the first four pudding-bundles are in use, the other four are to be kept in the mixture of decoction and milk placed over the fire when the earlier one's cool down, they are placed in the pan and the warm ones are taken out of it for use. The massage should be conducted without any appreciable interruption or break. Therefore, replacing the cold pudding-bundles with the hot ones should be as quick as possible.[29]

Position of the body

The patient should first be on the massage table in the (1) Sitting posture. After massage for sometime, he is to be made to lie on his (2) back and the massage should be continued in this position. Thereafter, he is to be made to lie on (3) The right side, again on his (4) back and then on the (5) left side, once again on his (6) back and finally he should revert back to the (7) erect sitting posture. Massage is done in all these seven various postures. In each of these postures, massage should be done for 15 minutes approximately. The time of therapy can be increased or decreased depending upon the general condition and strength of the patient and the disease he is suffering from. The physician has to assess the exact requirements of the patient.[30]

During massage, generally the mixture of decoction and milk, which is kept over the pan for boiling, gets completely used up, because the bundle of the puddings have to be frequently dipped into it. After massage, these bundles are to be opened and the remaining portion of the pudding is to be taken out. This is to be applied over the body of the patient and gently rubbed according to the procedure followed for massage. This should be done for about five minutes. Thereafter, the pudding remaining adhered to the skin of the patient should be scrapped out with the help of a thin but blunt spatula or knife. Traditionally, it is done with the help of a coconut leaf. The oil of the head is removed by gently wiping with the help of a dry towel. The scrapping of the pudding and wiping out of the oil from the head should be done gently in order to avoid production of heat by friction etc.

The head and the body, thus cleaned are to be anointed with medicated oils. The medicated oil to be used for this purpose should be according to the necessity of the patient and it is to be selected by the physician. Then the patient should be given bath.

Bath

For bathing, the water should be boiled by adding some medicinal herbs which are to be selected by the physician. After boiling the herbs should be filtered out and the water should be allowed to cool till it becomes luke warm. For head however, water should not be warm at all. The water to be used for washing the head should be of normal room temperature.

In order to remove excess oil from the body and the head, the flour of green gram or chick-pea should be rubbed. It is better if an attendant is employed for giving bath to the patient, because the patient himself may not be able to apply the above mentioned flour uniformly in all parts of his body.

After bath the patient should be wrapped with a cotton or woolen blanket depending upon the nature of the season and climatic conditions and should be made to take rest for about an hour. He should not be disturbed by noise or exposed to the sun, dust, storm, cold wind and smoke. It is better if the patient while lying down recites *Om* or *Gāyatrī mantra*. People of different religion can recite the holy scriptures of their respective faiths. The patient should not sleep during this time and light food can be given to him thereafter.[31]

Course of Therapy

The course of therapy varies depending up on the strength and nature of the disease the patient is suffering from. The therapy can be applied daily or on alternate for a period of 7 to 14 days at a stretch. The course of treatment has to be decided by the physician. Traditionally a course of this therapy may last 7,9,11 or 14 days. For every alternate therapy, the position of the body of the patient should be changed. Masseurs are of different types and in spite of all precautions, they may be putting different types of pressure while performing massage. Changing the posture of the body alternatively during alternative therapy, will eliminate this likely defect.

Benefits

This therapy endows several benefits to a healthy person and to a patient. This causes both oleation and simultaneous fomentation of the body. It makes the body supple, removes stiffness and swelling in joints and cures diseases caused by the aggravation of *vāta*. Once the channels of circulation are cleared of obstructions the blood circulation becomes better and it removes waste products from the body. It improves the complexion of the skin, increases *pitta* promotes digestion and restores vigour. It prevents excessive sleep but endows the person with sound sleep during night. This therapy is very effective in curing diseases of the nervous system chronic rheumatism, osteo arthritis, gout, emaciation of muscles in the limbs and cures diseases caused by the vitiation of the blood. It makes the body strong and sturdy with well -developed masculature. It promotes sharpness of the vision and the functions of other sensory organs. It is very effective for persons having insomnia, high blood pressure, diabetes and obstinate skin diseases. It prevents the process of aging, premature greying, of hair, baldness, appearances of wrinkles over the body and other ailments caused by the process of aging.

Restrictions

Some restrictions are required to be observed in respect of diet and regiments during the course of the therapy and for an equal number of days after the therapy.

Preparation of the patient

Once a week before the actual treatment begins, the patient should be given a daily dose of light laxative to keep his bowels clean. During the course of treatment and for an equal number of days thereafter the patient should take proper diet, drink and he should be free from physical as well as mental exertion.

Water for drinking and Bath

For the purpose of drinking water boiled with coriander, dry ginger, and cumin seeds should be used. After boiling water should be cooled and then given to the patient to drink. For bath and other cleaning purpose suluke warm water is recommended.

Conduct and Regimens

The patient should abstain from sexual intercourse. Even the thought of sex should not come to one's mind. Suppression of natural urges like excretion should be strictly prohibited. Nor should the patient undertake any strenuous physical exercise.

Diet

The patient during the course of the therapy and for an equal number of days thereafter, should take light food at regular intervals. The ingredients, which are in a liquid or semi-solid form, which are warm and which do not cause any burning sensation should be given to the patient. In addition to the quality it is essential to see that the patient takes food in appropriate quantities. After the patient feels satisfied with the food, he should not continue eating. As a general rule, half the capacity of the stomach should be filled with the solid, liquid, or semi-liquid food, 1/4th of the capacity of the stomach should be filled with water and the remaining 1/4th capacity of stomach should be kept empty.

Proper bowel movements is very important as far this treatment is concerned. Even during the course of therapy and thereafter, the physician should take care that the patient's bowels are moving freely .Other wise the therapy is not likely to produce the desired result.

Drinks

The patient should take water and milk, fruit juice and soup in adequate quantities during the course of therapy. Water boiled by adding coriander, dry ginger and cumin seeds should be cooled and kept ready in earthen pots for the convenience of the patient. The patient should take about 3-5 liters of water per day during and after the meals.

Proper sleep, clothing and light excise are also essential to attain good results. Excessive reading is prohibited because it may give rise to strain to the eyes. These precautions including diet, drinks and regimens should always be kept in view while administering different types of special massage therapies for the purpose of rejuvenation of the body and prevention as well as cure of obstinate and otherwise incurable diseases.[32]

Unfortunately such vital precautions are often overlooked in crass commercialism rampant in modern times in the name of health tourism. (See the illustrations at the end of the work)

Ilakkizhi (patrapoṭalasveda)

It is one of the most popular therapies in Kerala for the treatment of gout diseases especially for *pakṣavadha* (Paralysis). This therapy has another name *paccakkizhi*. It is a process by which the whole body is made to perspire by the application of certain medicinal puddings followed by massage. The commonly followed method is given below:

Preparation of Pudding

The leaves of the following plants namely *erukk* (Mudar), *āvaṇakk* (Castor), *muriñña* (Horse radish tree), *uññu* (Indian beech), *nīrmātaḷa* (Three leaved caper), *karinocci* (Five leaved chaste tree), *ummatt* (Thorn apple), *āṭaloṭaka* (Justica beddomei), *puḷi* (Tamarind), (Ripened leaf of) jack fruit tree and oil of *neem*, coconut scrapes (half a portion of a coconut), *lemon*, *śatakuppa* (Dill), *uluva* (Fenugreek), *kaṭuku* (Mustard), *induppu* (Ind salt) are required for this preparation. The proportion of ingredients for the preparation of pudding are according to the directions of physicians.

Firstly the leaves mentioned are cut into chips and then mixed with the scrapes of coconut, chips of lemon and the powder of Fenugreek etc. This mixture is boiled in Neem oil until it becomes red in colour. This should be divided into equal parts and made two boluses as in *piṇḍasveda*. The preparation of the patient and procedures of this therapy are the same as described in *piṇḍasveda*. But here only two attendants (nurses) are required. Traditionally a course of therapy may last for 7 to 14 days for half an hour each day. The course of therapy for each patient is to be decided by the physician.[33]

Nāraṅṅākkizhi

If the ingredients of *ilakkizhi* for the preparation of pudding are replaced with lemon chips, it is called *nāraṅṅākkizhi*. It is advisable to add the powders of Horse gram and, Fenugreek for better results. The procedures and other preparations are same in *ilakkizhi*.

This therapy is very effective in curing diseases of the osteo arthritis, emaciation of muscles in the limbs and shoulder pain.[34]

Poṭikkizhi

If the ingredients for the preparation of pudding in *ilakkizhi* are replaced by the powders of root of *āvaṇakku* (Castor), *koṭṭam* (Kutch), *candana* (Sandal), *cukku* (Dry ginger), *vayampu* (Sweet flag), *kaṭuku* (Mustard), *kuntirukkam*, (Indian olibanum tree), *devadāru* (Deodar) etc., it is called *poṭikkizhi*. The preparation and procedures are same as in *ilakkizhi*.

This therapy is very effective for the ailments connected with various gout diseases.[35] (See the illustrations at the end of the work)

Navadhānyakkizhi

If the ingredients for the preparation of the mixture in *poṭikkizhi* are replaced by the powders of the following namely *uzhunnu* (Black gram), *cerupayar* (Green gram), *eḷḷu* (Gingely), *mutira* (Horse gram), *āvaṇakkari* (Castor seed), *śatakuppa* (Dill), *navarayari* (Navara paddy), *uluva* (Fenugreek) etc. it called *navadhānyakkizhi*. For better results it is advisable to sink the boluses in coconut milk or cow milk during massage. The procedures, preparations and benefits are same as in *poṭikkizhi*.[36]

Nellikkāttaḷam

If *nellikkā* (embilica officianalis) and *rāmacca* (Vetiver) etc., are grinded in butter milk and made to paste form and put in the centre of the head according to the direction of the physician; It is called *nellikkāttaḷam*. Traditionally *nellikkā* (emblica officinalis) is only recommended for this therapy. The duration of this therapy is 7 to 14 days for an hour each day:- After that head is dried with a towel. Then *rāsnādicūrṇa* (medicated powder) is applied on the centre of the head and the head is covered with a boiled leaf.[37] (See the illustrations at the end of the work)

Urovasti

This therapy is effective for chest pain, gas trouble and difficulty in swallowing. Powder of black gram should be mixed with luke warm water and with that paste a covering is prepared around the thoracic region which enable the medicated oil not to flow from this region. Duration of this therapy is 7 to 14 days for 1.5 hrs. each day. The temperature of the medicated oil should be maintained by pouring necessary warm oil. The medicated oil for this therapy is selected by the physician.[38] (See the illustrations at the end of the work)

Kāyaseka (Pizhiccil)

For the treatment of diseases caused by the impairment of the functioning of the nervous system, this is perhaps the best therapy. It involves application of warm medicated oil over the body, according to a prescribed procedure, as a result of which the patient perspires uniformly.

Firstly the patient is made to sit over the wooden table specially made for this purpose. It is technically called as *Taila-droṇi*. The oil for this therapy varies according to the strength and nature of the patient. This is decided by the physician after examining the patient. A piece of clean cloth has to be tied on the head of the patient, at the level of the eyebrows, to prevent flowing down of the oil (to be poured) from the head to the eyes. This therapy is applicable to both healthy persons and patients. For healthy persons it causes rejuvenation of the body and helps in the preservation and production of positive health. In the case of patient it cures several diseases.

For a healthy person generally a mixture of the sesame oil and cow's ghee is used. Oil medicated by cooking with drugs for rejuvenating effects is also used in this therapy. The duration of the course of treatment may vary depending upon the nature of the disease and the physical as well as mental condition of the patient.[39]

The patient should be made to sit on the wooden table and four attendants should sit or stand-two on each side of the table. The medicated oil has to be made tolerably warm. With the help of pieces of cloth 50 cm X 50 cm in size the oil should be taken out of the oil pan and the cloth should be squeezed over the body of the patient by the masseurs with their hands. There is also another method for pouring oil by using specially prepared jars. The oil comes out uniformly from the narrow mouth of the jar. The oil is to be poured over the body of the patient with uniform and medium speed. It should be poured from a moderate height. First of all the medicated oil has to be applied over the head and then over the body. For application over the head the oil should be of room temperature and for the body, it should be lukewarm. Therefore the pouring should be performed gently. The pouring of the warm oil over the body should continue till the body starts perspiring on the fore-head chest and armpit. The attendants, while applying the oil in the above manner should at the same time, massage the body of the patient gently with their left hands. It should take very much about the temperature of the oil by the attendants because excessively hot oil may cause scald.

The process of massage is done all the seven postures described earlier to *piṇḍasveda (navarakkizhi)* therapy. Generally one and half hours to two hours time is required for one therapy. The pouring of the oil over the head should be done from a height of 8 cm from the level of the head. On the other parts height is 20 cm. The oil which is used for this therapy can be collected through the vessels, kept below the holes of the table and this oil can be repeatedly used for the same patient for three times more. Thereafter fresh oil should be used for the patient. If, however the patient can afford the expenditure, it is always better to use fresh oil every day.[40]

The patient at times feels completely exhausted after this therapy. In that case, he should be fanned and so cold water should be sprinkled over his body.

He should be made to take rest and then allowed to get up. Thereafter, the body should be massaged and excess oil from the body should be taken out with the help of a dry and clean towel. Thereafter, fresh oil is again applied to the head and the body and the flour of black gram or chick pea is sprinkled over the body and again cleaned to take out the excess of oil. Then the patient should be asked to take bath with water boiled with the leaves of medicinal plants. The water for the head should be of room temperature and water for the body should be lukewarm. Bath should be taken with the help of attendants. After the bath the patient is to be dressed with clean and dry cloths. Thereafter, he may be given water boiled with dried ginger and coriander to drink. If the patient feels hungry, he may be given some light and liquid food. The preparation should be boiled by adding digestive and carminative herbs. There will be some restrictions on his diet and regimen during the course of therapy and for the equal number of days thereafter. The patient should have absolute control over the body and mind and should avoid sexual intercourse altogether to get the best benefits of this therapy. He should be physically and mentally calm and quiet.

Duration of the treatment varies from person to person. It should be done daily or at an interval of one, two, three or four days. Generally one course involves administration of this therapy for 14 days.[41] (See the illustrations at the end of the work)

Thus it can be said that Kelala has contributed a lot in addition to the Āyurvedic materials mentioned in the authentic *samhitā* texts on Āyurveda.

References

1. Dr. C.K. Kareem, *Kerala and Her culture an Introduction*, State Editor Kerala Gazetters, TVM, 1971.

2. A. Sreedharan Menon, *A survey of Kerala history,* p.42.

3. Dr. N.V.K Varrier. '*Keralattinte Āyurveda Pāramparyam*' *Smaraṇikā,* Sree Sankaracharya Sanskrit University, p.124, 1999.

4. Raghava Varrier, Rajan Gurukkal, *Kerala Caritram*, Vallathol Vidyapeetham, Sukapuram, p.69. 1999,

5. K.N Ganesh, *Keralattinte innalekaḷ*, p.5. 1990.

6. *Kerala Caritram,* p.259.

7. *Ibid* p.257.

8. Dr.N.V.K Varrier *Smaraṇikā,* p.127.

9. Attupurath Impiccan Gurukkal, *Dhārākalpa* I-1

10. Moos. N. S, *Āyurvedic Treatments of Kerala.* p.11

11. *Idem*

12. *Dhārākalpa* I-22

    Kuryānnatvaparāhnakepi

    ca bhiṣagrātrau thatā secanam I

13. Vaida Bhagwan Dash, *Massage Therapy in Āyurveda,* p.65

14. *Ibid.* p. 67

15. *Ibid.* p. 67

16. Moos. N. S. *Āyurvedic Treatments of Kerala.* p.18

17. *Dhārākalpa* I-14

    Keśādīnāñca śauklyam klamamapi tanutām doṣakopam śirorug

    Bādhamojakṣayam tatkaracaraṇaparistodanam mūtradoṣam /

    Sandhīnām viślathatvam hṛdayarugaruci jāṭharāgneśca māndyam

    Dhātrītakrothadhārāharatiśirasivā karṇanetrāmayaugham //

18. Vaidya Bhagwan Dash, *Massage Therapy in Āyurveda* p. 68

19. *Ibid.* p. 69

20. *Dhārākalpa* I-9

   ūrdhvam keśabhuvo yāvadvamgulam

   Dhārayecciram āvaktranāsikak!edāt daśāṣṭau ṣaṭpalādiṣu

21. *Ibid*

22. *Aṣṭāṅgahṛdaya,* sūtrasthāna, 2-7,8

23. *Carakasamhitā,* sūtrasthāna, 2-15

24. *Suśrutasamhitā,* sūtrasthāna,5-3

25. Dr. Raghavan Thirumulppad, "Medical Science" *Technical Literature in Sanskrit.* p.151

26. Dash Bhagvan, *Massage Therapy in Āyurveda,* p.45

27. N. S. Moos, *Āyurvedic Treatments of Kerala,* p.28.

28. *Ibid*

29. *Dash* Bhagavan, *Massage Therapy in Āyurveda,* p. 48.

30. *Ibid* 49

31. *Ibid* 51

32. *Dhārākalpa,* 1. 10

33. Dr. K. Muraleedharan Pillai, '*Cila Saviśeṣa Āyurveda Cikitsakaḷ,*' *Vijñāna Kairaḷī,* June -2004, p.41.

34. *Ibid;*

35. *Ibid* p.42

36. *Ibid* p.43

37. *Ibid* p.44

38. *Ibid* p.44

39. *Ibid* 1. 11

40. Dash Bhagavan, *Massage theraphy in Āyurveda* "p. 80

41. *Dhārākalpa* 1.13.

Chapter 4

SOURCE BOOKS OF ĀYURVEDA IN KERALA - A SYNOPTIC SURVEY

The important work on the subject of medicine extant today are *Carakasamhitā, Suśrutasamhitā, Aṣṭāṅgasaṅgraha, Mādhavanidāna, Śārṅgadharasamhitā, Bhāvaprakāśasamhitā* and *Aṣṭāṅgahṛdaya. Samhitā* texts are authentic texts on Āyurveda which treat the important subject matter as a whole, emphasis being given to a particular branch of the science.[1] Most of the samhitā texts are not available in the original form now. It is surmised that they have undergone periodic revision by several hands until they attained their present form. From a study of text like *Carakasamhitā, Suśrutasamhitā* etc. it seems that there were other samhitās prior to those mentioned here, such as *Brahmasamhitā, Bhāradvājasamhitā, Dhanvatarasamhitā* etc. But either they were orally taught and studied and when writing came into vogue they were adapted and compiled into later *samhitās* or in due course of time they were lost, and now *Bhelasamhitā* and *Kāśyapasamhitā* are available only in fragments.

Among the extant texts, the *Carakasamhitā* by Caraka, the *Suśrutasamhitā* by Suśruta and *Aṣṭāṅgasaṅgraha* by Vāgbhaṭa are recognized as *Bṛhattrayī* or the Great Trio. They contains 120 chapters each. The authors of these texts are recognized as *Vṛddhatrayī. Mādhavanidāna*, by Mādhavācārya, *Śārṅgadharasamhitā* by Śārṅgadhara and *Bhāvaprakāśasamhitā* by Bhāvaprakāśa are recognized as *Laghutrayī* .Dr. Raghavan Thirumulppad points out that some scholars include *Aṣṭāṅgahṛdaya* or *Bhaiṣajyaratnāvalī* in *Laghutrayis* in place of *Mādhavanidāna*. [2]

Carakasamhitā

The *Carakasamhitā* is an enormous medical compilation, parts of which are entirely in verse, parts in prose alternating with verse, and parts simply in prose usually concluding with mnemonic verses. From the colophons at the end of each chapters in *Carakasamhitā,* it can be assumed that *Carakasamhitā,* which was originally composed by Agniveśa and was called *Agniveśasamhitā* was subsequently redacted by Caraka.[3]

Ityagniveśakṛte tantre carakapratisamskṛte

Sūtrasthāne dīrghamjīvatīyo nāma prathamo adhyāyaḥ

Even this redacted version is not available in its entirety now. Out of 120 chapters, about 41 chapters were missing and subsequently added by a fourth century scholar named Dṛḍhabala. This is evident from the following passage in *Carakasamhitā:*

asmin saptadaśādhyāyāḥ kalpaḥ siddhaya eva ca nāśādyante 'gniveśasya tantre carakasamskṛte tānetān kapilabali śeṣān dṛḍhabalo 'karot tantrasyās yamahārthasyapūraṇārtham yathātatham. 4

The seventeen chapters belongs to *kalpa* and *siddhi* chapters of the redacted version of *Agniveśasamhitā* by Caraka missed and later on subsequently added by Kapilabali and Dṛḍhabala for the completion of the work.

Modern scholars have different views regarding the date of *Carakasamhitā,* ranging from 6 B.C. to I A.D.[5] Dr. Raghavan Thirumulpad points out that Caraka belonged to 2 B.C. on the ground that Caraka was a court physician of Kaniska.[6] However the text available now redacted finally by Drdhabhala might have belonged to 1. A.D..

Carakasamhitā contains 120 (or, containing the sub-chapters on rasayana and *vajikarana,*126) chapters in all. These are arranged in eight books, namely;

1. *Sūtrasthāna,* discussing in 30 chapters the history, general principles, theoretical basis etc of modern medicine.

2. *Nidānasthāna,* intended to discuss in Eight chapters the causes of various diseases and their symptoms.

3. *Vimānasthāna*, discussing in eight chapters a wide range of assorted topics, like the nature and qualities of matter, the process of transformation within the body of various natural substance consumed, the methodology of medical science, codes of conduct of the medical practitioners etc.

4. *Śarīrasthāna*, intended to discuss in eight chapters mainly anatomy and embryology, though as a matter of fact the chapters often disgress into metaphysics, ethics etc., also

5. *Indriyasthāna*, discussing in 12 chapters various questions among which those concerning diagnosis and prognosis are prominent.

6. *Cikitsāsthāna,* discussing mainly therapeutics though also a great deal of dietics and pharmacology in 30 chapters in one version (containing the sub chapters of the first two chapters. In another version (or, containing the sub chapters of the first two chapters, 36 in all)).

7. *Kalpasthāna*, containing 12 comparatively brief chapters, evidently supplementing the pharmacopoeia of the earlier books.

8. *Siddhisthāna* containing 12 chapters on enema, purgation, urinary diseases etc. mainly supplementing what is discussed in the other books.

The text as a whole is full of repetitions and digressions. It also describes debates and disputes among various authorities on questions of basic theoretical importance.[7] What is highly interesting, is that according to the text such debates are extremely useful for expanding the mental horizon of the physicians.[8] What is remarkable, however, is that, in spite of the awareness of the differences among the different schools of medicine, the text insists that there are certain conclusions essential for medical science as such. The text calls these *sarva-tantra-siddhānta* or conclusions unanimously accepted by all schools of medicine.

tatra sarvatantrasiddhānto nāma tasmin tasmin sarvasmin tantre tat tat prasiddham, yadā santi nidānāni, santi vyādhayaḥ, santi siddhi upāyaḥ sādhyānām iti. [9]

Among these (conclusions) those are called unanimously admitted ones which have reputation in each and every treatise on the subject (viz medicine).

Such are: there are causes; there are diseases, there are ways of curing the curable diseases.

It is interesting to note that at the time of Caraka himself there were fake physicians. So in his *Samhitā*, Caraka advices the doctors as follows which is some what similar to the Hipocratic oath.

> *nārthārtham nāpi kāmārthamatha bhūtadayām prati*
>
> *vartate yaścikitsāyām sa sarvamativartate*
>
> *kurvate ye tu vṛtyartham cikitsāpaṇyavikrayam*
>
> *te hitvā kāñcanam rāsim pāmsurāśimupāsate*
>
> *dāruṇai kṛṣyamāṇānām gadairvaivasvatakṣayam*
>
> *chitvā vaivasvatān pāśān jīvitam yaḥ prayacchati*
>
> *dharmārthadātā sadṛśastasya nehopalabhyate*
>
> *na hi jīvitadānāddhi dānamanyad viśiṣyate*
>
> *paro bhūtadayādharma iti matvā cikitsayā*
>
> *vartate yaḥ sa siddhārthaḥ sukhamatyantamaśnute.* [10]

Among the physicians, he surpasses all who practices medicine neither for the sake of money nor for the sake of sensual gratification in any form, but is motivated only by the compassion for living beings. Those who, as a source of income, want to sell medical skill as any other commodity, appear to run after a leap of dust, overlooking the real hoard of gold. Compared to the physician who cuts off the noose of death and brings back to life those who are being dragged by fierce diseases towards death, nobody confers greater blessings moral or materials to the human beings. One who practices the healing art with compassion for the living beings as the noblest of all duties is a person who really fulfills his mission and thereby gets entitled to the highest form of happiness.

In short *Carakasamhitā* being an authentic text on *kāyacikitsā* touches each and every aspect of human life. It also deserves special mention that *Carakasamhitā* contains reference to six hundred types of medicines.

Suśrutasamhitā

Suśrutacaryā composed the original *samhitā* in his name. He was considered to be a disciple of Dhanvatari. Like *Carakasamhitā*, it is also written in classical

Sanskrit, partly in verse and partly in prose. The text available now is edited by a Nāgārjuna. Nāgārjuna not only redacted *Suśrutasamhitā* but also added *uttaratantra* to it. *Suśrutasamhitā* contains reference to 650 varieties of medicines and 121 types of surgical instruments. It also mentions 300 kinds of surgeries and also directions for 42 different ways of doing it.[11] Even Caraka himself states that physicians of Dhanvantari school are experts in surgery.

tatra dhānvantarīyāṇamadhikāraḥkriyāvidhau /

vaidyānām kṛtayogyānām vyatha śodhanaropaṇe.[12]

Caraka and Suśruta combined together represent Āyurveda in its fullness. What is wanting in one is supplied by the other.

yadi carakamadhīte taddhruvam suśrute hi

praṇigaditagadānām nāmamātrepi bāhyaḥ

atha carakavihīnaḥ prakriyāyāmakhinnaḥ

kimiva khalu karotu vyādhitānām varākaḥ //[13]

He (physician) who reads only the Caraka (*samhitā*) is deprived of even the names of the diseases which are described by Suśruta (*samhitā*) etc. and who is devoid of (not studied) Caraka (*samhitā*) becomes inefficient in giving treatment. What good can such an unintelligent man can do to the patient.

Literature is the reflection of society of its times; the importance given to Suśruta and Caraka can be inferred from *Naiṣadhīyacarita of Śrīharṣa* :

Kanyāntaḥpurabodhanāya yadadhīkārānnadoṣā nṛpam

dvau mantripravaraśca tulyamagadamkāraśca tāvūcatuḥ

devākarṇaya suśrutena carakasyoktena jāne 'khilam

syādasyā naladam vinā na dalane tāpasya ko 'pi kṣamaḥ. //[14]

The doctor and the ministers alike, having the privilege to enter into the Princess's chamber, reported the matter thus: "Listen, my Lord there is no other medicine than *naladam* (a pun which could mean a medicinal herb called *naladam* and the union with king *Nalada*,)at once to cure the body's *tāpa* (sickness and love sickness at once) according to the ancient physicians Caraka and Suśruta (and as reported by the 'Caraka' or the spy.)

Modern scholars have different views regarding the time Date of *Suśrutasamhitā* ranging from 4 BC to 4AD.[15] Dr. Raghavan Thirumulpad observes after examining the language and subject matter that it may be later than *Carakasamhitā,* and the date is supposed to be 1 B.C.. The text available now with the redaction of Nagarjuna is seems to be composed in 4 A.D. [16]

The main body of *Suśrutasamhitā* contains 120 chapter arranged in five books. These are

(1) *sūtrasthāna*, discussing chapters in 46 chapters various topics inclusive of the general principle of medicine, the use and construction of surgical appliances, practice of surgery, cauterization.

(2) *nidānasthāna* – discussing in 16 chapters mainly the causes of diseases

(3) *śarīrasthāna*, discussing in 10 chapters mainly anatomy, embryology and the technique of dissection.

(4) *Cikitsāsthāna*, discussing in 40 chapters therapeutic techniques

(5) *Kalpasthāna*, discussing mainly toxicology in eight chapters.

It is also note worthy that this text also contains repetitions and certain unscientific ways of treatment, particularly in the treatment of infants and psychological disorders.[17]

Aṣṭāṅgasaṅgraha

It is an authoritative treatise on Āyurveda consisting of 150 chapters. As pointed out, its author Vāgbhaṭa is regarded as one of the *Vṛddhattrayī*. It is a compilation of information of the *Aṣṭāṅgas,* the eight branches of Āyurveda in one text. As before compiling of *Aṣṭāṅgasaṅgraha*, each of these eight branches had its own separate books, written by sages but their study was difficult. The object of this work according to Vāgbhaṭa is thus;

Each one of the texts written by them (sages) by itself does not describe all the diseases, to study all the texts would require a whole lifetime; since many things are common to all texts. Hence this text has been written by collecting only the essence from all; it is devoid of textual blemishes, confines only to the three pillars (of medical science) viz. *hetu* (knowledge of causes of diseases) *liṅga* (symptomatology) and *auṣadha* (therapeutics), it explains many hidden, doubtful and contrary points; is composed so as to be suitable to the present age, with emphasis on *kāyacikitsā* (inner medicine) since it is difficult for understanding and pervades all other branches; there is not a single syllable here which is not supported by the scriptures, change in the mode of composition is done for the sake of brevity only and nothing else. [18]

The 150 chapters of *Aṣṭāṅgasaṅgraha* are comprised under six chapters. They are as follows:

1.	*sūtrasthāna*	40 chapters
2.	*śarīrasthāna*	12 chapters
3.	*nidānasthāna*	16 chapters
4.	*cikitsāsthāna*	24 chapters
5.	*kalpasthāna*	8 chapters
6.	*uttarasthāna*	50 chapters
		150 chapters in all

Sūtrasthāna describes the basic doctrines, principles of health, prevention of diseases, diet articles, food habits, causes of diseases and methods of treatments.

Śarīrasthāna describes the evolution and composition of the universe, human embryology, anatomy, physiology, physical and psychological temperaments — dreams etc.

Nidānasthāna describes the causes, signs, symptoms, pathogenesis, prognosis etc of major diseases.

Cikitsāsthāna describes the methods of treatment, medicines, diet, care of the patient etc of all diseases pertaining to *kayacikitsa* (inner medicine)

Kalpasthāna deals with principles of pharmacy, weights and measures, method of preparing purificatory recipes etc.

Uttarasthāna, the final section, has 51 chapters forming one third of the total chapters. The distribution of contents are given as follows:

1.	*bālacikitsā* (Pediatrics)		5 chapters
2.	*grahacikitsā* (demonology)		5 chapters
3.	*ūrdhvāṅgacikitsā*		
	a)	*netrarogacikitsā* (ophthalmology)	10 chapters
	b)	*karṇarogacikitsā* (otology)	2 chapters
	c)	*nāsārogacikitsā* (rhinology)	2 chapters

<table>
<tr><td>d)</td><td>Mukharogacikitsā (treatment of lips, teeth, gums, tongue, palate and throat)</td><td>2 chapters</td></tr>
<tr><td>e)</td><td>Śiroroga (treatment of head and scalp)</td><td>2 chapters</td></tr>
<tr><td>4.</td><td>śalyacikitsā (surgery)</td><td>11 chapters</td></tr>
<tr><td>5.</td><td>daṃṣṭrā / viṣacikitsā (toxicology)</td><td>9 chapters</td></tr>
<tr><td>6.</td><td>jara / rasāyana (rejuvenation)</td><td>2 chapters</td></tr>
<tr><td>7.</td><td>vṛṣa / vājīkaraṇa (virilification)</td><td>1 chapter</td></tr>
<tr><td></td><td></td><td>51 chapters</td></tr>
</table>

The text consists of both prose and verse. Some chapters have prose and verse both, while some others have only either of them. The language and style of composition are archaic and tough. A deep study of *Aṣṭāṅgasaṅgraha* may reveal many blemishes such as repetition of same subject both in prose and verse, elaborate description of religious rites and ceremonies, unsequential placement of topic etc. have got into the text, contrary to the assertion of the author.[19] This leads us to presume lack of adequate attention of the author at the time of compilation.

Author

In the *uttarasthāna* of *Aṣṭāṅgasaṅgraha* there is a reference to the author's personal details --

> *bhiṣagvaro vāgbhaṭa ityabhūnme*
>
> *pitāmaho nāmadharo 'smi yasya /*
>
> *suto 'bhavattasya ca simhagupta-*
>
> *stasyapyaham sindhuṣu labdhajanmā //*
>
> *samadhigamya guroravalokitāt*
>
> *gurutarācca pituḥ pratibhān mayā*
>
> *subahubheṣajaśāstravilokanāt*
>
> *suvihito 'ṅga vibhāgavinirṇayaḥ //* [20]

There was a great physician by name Vāgbhaṭa, who was my grandfather, and I bear his name, from him was born Simhagupta and I am from him (Simhagupta) born in the land of Sindhu. Having acquired sound knowledge from Avalokita the preceptor and even more from the wisdom of my father and after studying a large number of texts of medical science this treatise has been written suitably classified (in to branches, sections, chapters etc.)

From the above information it can be seen that there is a reference to Avalokita, the chief god of Mahāyāna Buddhism as his preceptor. This is suggestive of the religion he belonged to. Apart from these, he has not furnished any other information. The only information available about him is from the writing of the later authors. But from the study based on the available sources also, nothing definite can be said on this matter.

Preceptor

Vāgbhaṭa mentioned Avalokita as his preceptor. Avalokiteśvara is the chief divinity of Mahāyāna sect of Buddhism. He is the Bodhisatva (future Buddha) and was being worshiped since the days of emporer Aśoka. Idols of god begin to appear from the Gupta period (300-550 AD).[21] If this god is taken as the preceptor, then it will be more a religious tradition and so only nominal. If, however, Avalokita is taken to mean a person of that name, it would suggest that he belonged to the Buddhist religion.

However it was a name of person named Avalokita, then there should be some evidence at least. So far no such evidence for the existence of a scholar (Buddhist) of that name has come to light.

Meanwhile it is interesting to note that Niścalakara calls Vāgbhaṭa as Śaunakaśiṣya- pupil of Śaunaka.[22] Jejjaṭa the disciple of Vāgbhaṭa also has mentioned Vāgbhaṭa as a follower of following Śaunaka: *saunakamatam anuavadatā vāgbhaṭena* (*Vāgbhaṭa approving / substaining the opinion of Śaunaka*). No other information is available about Śaunaka.[23]

Moreover Vāgbhaṭa also states that he learnt much from his father Simhagupta. That Simhagupta was a scholar and also a reputed physician can be guessed by the honorofic title *Vaidyapati* (king of physicians) attached to his name in colophon of some manuscript of *Aṣṭāṅgahṛdaya* at the end of every chapter. [24] Soḍhala (12-13 AD) in his work refers to a medicinal formula compounded by Simhagupta.[25]

Disciples

Jejjeṭa in the colophon of his commentary on *Carakasamhitā* styles himself as *Vāgbhaṭaśiṣya* the disciple of Vāgbhaṭa: *iti vāgbhaṭaśiṣyajajjaṭasya kṛtau nirantarapada vyākhyāyām.*[26]

Nīlamegha (9 AD) in his work *Tantrayuktivicāra* offers obeisance to Vāgbhaṭa and says Indu and Jejjeṭa are his desciples.[27] This verse in course of time became popular and created the belief that both Jejjata and Indu are pupils of Vāgbhaṭa.

P.V Sharma disagrees with the above views. He observes thus: 1) Jejjata calls his teacher by his name without any reverential epithets which is contrary to the custom prevalent, Then 2) Jejjata can be placed in the 9th century, two centuries later than Vāgbhaṭa. With regard to Indu, the objection is again the date, Indu can only be placed in 13 AD and not earlier.[28] Srikantamurthy in his introduction to the text *Aṣṭāṅgasaṅgraha* disagree with P.V Sarma as to the view made by him about *Jajjata*. K.R Srikanthamurthy points out that one cannot disbelieve the statement made by Jejjata himself who was a scholar of great merit, who wrote erudite commentaries on the works of Caraka, Suśruta and also Vāgbhaṭa which are quoted by later commentaries reverently. Moreover it seems probable that Jejjata belonged to Kashmir and might have traveled to the nearby Sindh to study under Vāgbhaṭa. There are divergent opinions regarding his date ranging from 6th to 9th century AD. Meulenbeld expresses the value that Jajjeṭa's date may be about 600 AD. (the age in which Vāgbhaṭa lived). So K.R Srikantha Murthy concludes that Jejjata was a disciple of Vāgbhaṭa.[29]

Religion

The religion to which Vāgbhaṭa belonged is another topic of debate since plenty of references are found to both Hinduism and Buddhism in his Work, *Aṣṭāṅgasaṅgraha*. Taking advantage of this one set of modern Āyurveda scholars assert that he was a follower of Hinduism while another set assert that he was a Buddhist. Some important points of both religions are furnished here.

Hinduism (Purāṇic)

The evidences in support of the claim that Vāgbhaṭa followed Hinduism include his mention of gods like Brahmā, Dakṣa, Indra, Aśvins, Rudra, Viṣṇu, Soma,

Sūrya, Durgā, Kārtikeya, Vināyaka etc. worship of cows and brāhmaṇas, conduct of *Yajña* and offering gifts to gods, study of the Vedas, chanting of hymns, observance of *Ātharvaṇic* rites, pilgrimage to holy places etc, legends connected with origin of diseases eg. dakṣayajña, rudrakopa, vīrabhadrajanana, creation of bālagrahas by Rudra to protect Skanda, spiders born from the sweat of Viśvāmitra by his wrath against Vasiṣṭha, non prohibiting of meat and wine and the like.

Buddhism

The evidences in support of the claim that Vāgbhaṭa followed Buddhism include his obeisance to Buddha specifically at the beginning of the text, modes of addresses such as *Bhaiṣajyaguru, Vaidūrya prabharāja* to Buddha only; The mention of gods like Avalokita, Ārya Tārā, Praṇāśabarī, Aparājitā Maṇibhadra, Yakṣa, etc., prescribing the chanting of *Dhāraṇis* (protective hymns) like *Mayūrī, Mahāmayūrī* and *Bījamantras* (secret syllables) before administering medicine and also during treatments, mention of four *Āryasatya*, four kinds of death, worship of Bodhi tree, remembering Śāsta before sleep, adopting the *madhyamamārga* (middle path) in all activities etc; acceptance of the work of Vāgbhaṭa (*Aṣṭāṅgahṛdaya* especially) as a scared text in Buddhist countries like Tibet and China. [30]

From the above it becomes clear that Vāgbhaṭa has shown equal reverence to both religions. Nothing definite can be said on this matter. Whether he is a Buddhist or the follower of Hinduism. There is no dispute over the fact that his contribution to Āyurveda is great.

Other Works of Vāgbhaṭa

1. *Aṣṭāṅgahṛdaya* – it is the masterpiece of Vāgbhaṭa followed by Kerala physicians. A detail account of the text is given in the next chapter.

2. *Aṣṭāṅgāvatāra* – Jejjaṭa in his commentary on *Carakasamhitā* has mentioned a text by name *Aṣṭāṅgāvatāra*.[31] Aruṇadatta in his commentary quotes a verse from that and says that it is the work of the author of *Aṣṭāṅgahṛdaya*.[32] Nothing more about this text is known.

3. *Madhya Vāgbhaṭa / Madhyasamhitā*

   Niścalakara in his commentary on Cakradatta and Śivadāsa sen in his commentary on *Aṣṭāṅgahṛdaya* have quoted many verses and some prose passages from another text which they have called as *Madhya Vāgbhaṭa* or *Madhyasamhitā* (the middle text of Vāgbhaṭa). These verses resembles very much those of both *Aṣṭāṅgasaṅgraha* and *Aṣṭāṅgahṛdaya* but do not belong to either. This makes it imperative for us to accept the existence of this intermediary text written by Vāgbhaṭa.

4. *Aṣṭāṅganighaṇṭu* – This is a small book of about 408 verses, being a lexicon of synonyms of drugs mentioned in the *gaṇas* (drug groups) in *Aṣṭāṅgasaṅgraha* as the author says in the beginning of the book. But the colophon at the end of the Manuscript reads as "thus ends *Aṣṭāṅganighaṇṭu* of *Aṣṭāṅgahṛdayasamhitā* written by Bāhaṭācārya.[33]

   In one of the manuscripts, at its commencement there is a prayer to Lord Śiva, in addition to the invocatory verse present in *Aṣṭāṅgahṛdaya*. The practice of preparing a *nighaṇṭu* (lexicon) of drugs in ancient times is confirmed by the existence of such a lexicon attached to *Suśrutasamhitā*.[34]

   P.V Sharma the editor of the book opines that it is the work of a person different from the author at *Aṣṭāṅgahṛdaya* and places him in the 8th AD.[35]

5. *Rasaratnasamuccaya* – This is a text dealing with *Rasaśāstra* (Iatro chemistry) and treatment of diseases using mercurical and metallic compounds along with vegetable drugs. At the commencement of the text it is mentioned that Vāgbhaṭa, son of Simhagupta is the author.[36] But it stands in no comparison in the nature of the contents, composition and standard either with *Aṣṭāṅgasaṅgraha or Aṣṭāṅgahṛdaya*. Based on internal and external evidences it has been concluded that its author is a psudo-Vāgbhaṭa a person who has concealed his real name and passed on the book in the name of an earlier celebrity and this book can be assigned to 13th AD and not earlier.[37] So neither he nor his book is taken into consideration in the discussions concerning Vāgbhaṭa, author of *Aṣṭāṅgasaṅgraha*.

The problem of two Vāgbhaṭa

There is a controversy among scholars that whether there is one Vāgbhaṭa or two. One set of scholars believe that they are two and another favour the identity of the both.

Vāgbhaṭas are two

According to this Vāgbhaṭa son of Simhagupta and grandson of Vāgbhaṭa is the author of *Aṣṭāṅgasaṅgraha* while the author of *Aṣṭāṅgahṛdaya* is a different person having the same name. The following points are the basics for this view.[38]

1. Commentators such as those of Ḍalhaṇa, Vijayarakṣita, Śrīkaṇṭhadatta, Hemādri, Śivadāsa sena, etc. have quoted verses of *Aṣṭāṅgasaṅgraha* by the name 'as from *Vṛddhavāgbhaṭa*' and verses of *Aṣṭāṅgahṛdaya* by the name as from *Laghuvāgbhaṭa* / *Svalpavāgbhaṭa* or (simply) Vāgbhaṭa to show distinctness of two persons.

2. Many of the dissimilarities are seen between the two texts, such as nature and style of composition, scientific doctrines and practices, religious and social customs etc. All these go to prove different authorship only.[39]

3. Both the texts being almost of the same size, no scholar would waste his time and energy to write more than one book on the same subject.

    Modern scholars agree with the above view are P.Cordier, J.Jolly, A.F.R Hoerule, A.B. Keith, M.Winternitz, G.M Mukhopadhyaya, P.K Gode, P.V Sharma etc. Hoernle designated the author of *Aṣṭāṅgasaṅgraha* as Vāgbhaṭa –I and the author of *Aṣṭāṅgahṛdaya* as Vāgbhaṭa – II

Vāgbhaṭa is one

The following arguments are adduced in support of this view.

1. Earlier commentaries like Candrānanda, Indu, Aruṇadatta, Niścalakara, Bhaṭṭanarahari, etc. held this view.

2. The author's own statement at the end of the *Aṣṭāṅgahṛdaya* is that it is born out of *Aṣṭāṅgasaṅgraha* and written separately for the benefit of the less studious.[40]

3. Non – mention of author's name in *Aṣṭāṅgahṛdaya* is intentional, since the author is sure that anybody who reads it will certainly take it to be another work of the author of *Aṣṭāṅgasaṅgraha*. Since his personal whereabouts are furnished in that, it is not necessary to repeat it again.

4. Incorporation of verses without any change from one text to another also proves common authorship.

5. Similarities between the two texts are greater than dissimilarities. Epitomisation of an earlier elaborate and difficult text is apparent in *Aṣṭāṅgahṛdaya*.

6. There are many instance in ancient times in India that the same author writing more than one book on the same subject, the first one usually being big and tough, while the subsequent ones smaller and easier.

Modern scholars who subscribe to this view are T. Rudraparāśara, Bhagawat simhaji, Gaṇanāth sen, Haridatta Śāstry, N.S. Moos, Hariśāstry Paraḍkar, D.C Baṭṭācārya, Nandakishore sharma, Atridevagupta, C. Vogel, G.J Mulenbeld and Dr. Raghavan Thirumulpad.

K.R Srikanthamurthy critically analyses the above two views and arrives at a conclusion that Vāgbhaṭa is one and the same. He puts forward following arguments to prove this.[41]

1) If the author of *Aṣṭāṅgahṛdaya* is considered as the grandson of the *Aṣṭāṅgasaṅgraha*, then we have to accept the existence of another Simhagupta (the second) also, So far no reference indicating such a lineage has come to light.

2) No scholar capable of writing a book will copy the verses verbatim from a book of another author even though he might be descendent of the same family; in such a case he would certainly announce his family reputation at least with great pride. Since there is no such mention in *Aṣṭāṅgahṛdaya* it is impossible to think of any person other than Vāgbhaṭa as its author. A study of the text indicates that much gap of time cannot be envisaged between them. This fact also negates the assumption of a second or third generation of author for *Aṣṭāṅgahṛdaya*.

3) Difference on some major and minor points of scientific doctrines, practices, social costumes etc seen between the two texts can be

understood to have occurred not due to different authors but due to following reasons.

a)   Lack of attention – at the time of preparing *Aṣṭāṅgasaṅgraha* the author devoted all his attention to collection of material from large number of texts and compiling these and so could not have paid much attention to evaluate these.

b)   Changes in the social, religious and politics conditions taking place quickly after the disappearance of the Gupta empire had its effect on all literary works including medical sciences.

The above view seems to be more logical because when one go through the *uttarasthāna* of *Aṣṭāṅgahṛdaya* it can be see that there are some unsatisfactory comments implied by the author probably about the lack of attention of physicians to his former work *Aṣṭāṅgasaṅgraha*.[42]

Laghutrayīs

Mādhavanidāna

It has another name called *Rugviniścaya;* It was composed by Mādhavācārya of 8 A D. At the end of the work there is a colophon thus: Śrīmādhavendukarātmajena.[43] From this one can infer that his name is Mādhava and his father's name is Indukara. Scholars are of different opinion about his date. Keith places him to 8th or 9th century A.D.[44]

The text gives emphasis to the *nidana* (cause) of all diseases mentioned in *Carakasamhitā* and *Suśrutasamhitā*. The text begins with *pañcalakṣananidāna* and ends with *snāyukanidāna* in 74 chapters. *Mādhavācārya* gives *nidānas* (causes) of diseases also from his experience also in his text; So there is a popular saying that *nidāne mādhavaḥ śreṣṭha iti [Mādhava excells everybody in the area of causes (of diseases)]*.

Śārṅgadharasamhitā

It was written by Śārṅgadhara of 14 A.D. A feature of the text is the systematic arrangement of the subject matter and its preciseness. It is considered to be a hand - book of practicing physicians. The text opens with the verse.

prasiddhayogo munibhiḥ prayuktaḥ

cikitsakair yaḥ bahuśo 'nubhūtāḥ /

vidhīyate śārṅgadhareṇa teṣām

susamgrahaḥ sajjanarañjanāya // [45]

The popular recipes found out (prepared) by sages and attested by physicians through their experiences are abridged here by Śārṅgadhara for the appreciation of the scholars.

The book is remarkable for the scientific treatment of the topics in it. The process of respiration mentioned in it is a case in point :

nābhisthaḥ prāṇapavanaḥ spṛṣṭvā hṛtkamalāntaram

kaṇṭhādbahirviniryāti pātum viṣṇupadamṛtam /

pītvācāmbarapīyūṣam punarāyāti vegataḥ

prīṇayan dehamakhilam jīvam ca jaṭharānilam // [46]

The air in the abdomen goes to the heart and then get and through the neck for drinking *viṣṇupadāmṛtam* (may be oxygen), after drinking *ambarapīyūṣa* (oxygen) return back and animate the whole body and digestive process.

It is also stated here that life exists as long as this process continues. When this cases death occurs.

śarīraprāṇayorevam samyogādāyurucyate

kālena tadviyogācca pañcatvam kathyate budhaiḥ // [47]

Scholars speak thus: When body and *prāṇavāyu* (air which sustains may be oxygen) are combined together life exists and when they separated death occurs.

The text is divided into three *khaṇḍas. Pūrva, madhya* and *uttara*. It has 2600 *ślokas* in total distributed in 32 chapters. The *pūrvakhaṇḍa* consists of seven chapters, *uttarakhaṇḍa* consists of 13 chapters and *madhyakhaṇḍa* consists of 12 chapters.

Bhāvaprakāśasamhitā

It was composed by *Bhāvaprakāśamiśra* of 16th A.D. The text begins with the verse.

śrīpatipadaprasādāśībhirbhumidevānām

Bhāvaprakāśanāmnā grantho 'yam paṭhyatām sarvaiḥ /

śāstrejāḍyāntakāram

Praśamayitumimam samvidhatte prakāśam // [48]

Let all read this work named *Bhāvaprakāśa* composed by the blessings of Viṣṇu and other deities......... This is meant to remove the (darkness of) ignorance.

The text is divided into three *khaṇḍas. Pūrva, uttara* and *madhyama. Pūrvakhaṇḍa* contains seven *prakaraṇas*. It is again divided into *pūrva* and *uttara*, consisting of the first six *prakaraṇas* and one *prakaraṇa* respectively. The portion of the *pūrvaprakaraṇa* begins with *harītakyādivarga* upto *anekārthanāmavarga* is popularly known as *Bhāvaprakāśanighaṇṭu. Madhyakhaṇḍa* is again divided into four *adhikaraṇas. Phiraṅgaroga* (syphillis) brought to India by Portuguese is described in it with effective treatment. *Uttarakhaṇḍa* is also divided into two *adhikaraṇas*; *vājīkaraṇa* and *rasāyana* respectively.

Other works on Āyurveda

1. *Kāśyapasamhitā* - is the only available source on *Kaumārabhṛtya*, which is in the form of compilations of the preaching of god Kāśyapa by his disciple Vṛddha Jīvaka. The text available now is edited by Rajaguru Hemaraja Sharma of Nepal in 1938. The text contains only one fourth or even less than what it would have been in its original form. The text is divided into 120 chapters. [49] The other divisions are like *Carakasamhitā.*

   aṣṭau sthānāni vācyāni tato 'tastantramucyate /

   adhyāyānām śatam vimśam yo 'dhīte satu pāragaḥ //

2. *Bhelasamhitā* — composed by Bhela is available only in fragments. Bhela is considered to be a disciple of Punarvasu Ātreya. The subject matter mentioned in it are similar to those in *Carakasamhitā*. Bhela does not get proper attention because of his style. The text is also divided into 120 chapters. Vāgbhaṭa at one place refer to Bhela. *Bhelādyaḥ kim na paṭhyante* [50] which conforms to the good presentation and acceptability of that text.

3. *Harītasamhitā* — This work is written by one Hārīta who is considered to be a contemporary of Agniveśa and a disciple of Ātreya. But the text available now is not so old and hence it is not authentic.

4. *Nāvanītakam* – It is a part of 'Bower manuscript' discovered by a British army official named Bower from Kashgar in central Asia. Among the seven manuscripts recovered three deal with medicine. The important one is *Nāvanītakam* which contains *mahāmayūravidyā*, *mātaṅgavidyā* and *laśunakalpam* in addition to the topics described in *Carakasamhitā* and *Suśrutasamhitā*. It was composed during Gupta period. The original text is kept at Oxford University.

5. *Siddhayoga* or *Vṛndamādhavagrantha* - It was composed by one Vṛndamādhava of 9 A.D

6. *Cikitsāsamhitā* or *Cakradatta* and *Dravyaguṇasaṅgraha*. Both these works were composed by Cakrapāṇidatta of 10 A.D.

7. *Cikitsāsārasamhitā* or *Vaṅgasenagrantha* – It was composed by one Vaṅgasena of 12 A.D.

8. *Rasaratnasamuccaya* - It was an important *rasa* text composed by one Vāgbhaṭa of 13 A.D. Mercury, Sulphur, Iron, Silver, Gold and other metals are the drugs used in *Rasacikitsā*. There is a dispute over the authorship of *Rasaratnasamuccaya*; whether it is the work of the author of *Aṣṭāṅgasaṅgraha* and *Aṣṭāṅgahṛdaya*. To differentiate him from the original Vāgbhaṭa the author is called *Rasavāgbhaṭa* by scholars.

9. *Vīrasimhāvalokana* – The work was composed by king Vīrasimha in 1383 A.D. It contains topic like astrology, law and medicine.

10. *Kaumārabhṛtyam* – It was composed by Pṛthvīmalla in 1400 A.D..

11. *Rasaratnākara* – It was composed by Nityānanda of 15 A.D.

12. *Rasendramaṅgala or Rasaratnākara* – It was composed by Nāgārjuna. Only four chapters are available now.

13. *Āyurvedasaukhyam* or *Toṭalānandam* – It was composed by Raja Toṭarmal who was the minister of Akbar the mughal King.

14. *Rasahṛdayatantra*–It was composed by Govindapāda, the teacher of Śaṅkarācārya.

15. *Vaidyajīvanam* - It was composed by Lolimbaraja of 17 A.D. It contains many practical preparations (*yogas*)

16. *Yogaratnākara* – It is an anonymous work of 17 A.D.

17. *Gadanigraha* – It was composed by Sodhala of 18 A.D.

18. *Prayogāmṛtam* – It was composed by vaidyacintamani of 18 A.D.

19. *Vaidyāmṛtam* – It was composed by Narayana of 18 A.D.

20. *Bhaiṣajyaratnāvali* – It is a manual of diseases and treatments.

It is a popular work composed by Govindadas of 18 A.D.

References

1. Dr. Raghavan Thirumulppad, "Medical science", *Technical literature in Sanskrit*, p.65

2. Dr. Raghavan Thirumulppad, *Āyurvedaparicayam*, Nagarjuna Publications, p.125.

3. *Carakasamhitā*. I -Concluding colophon

4. *Ibid*, 4-30

5. *Śāstram indiayil*, p.19

6. *'Medical science'*, Op.cit. .p 69

7. *Carakasamhitā* I –12,25,26 etc

8. *Ibid* III – 8-15

9. *Ibid* III –8-37

10. *Ibid* VI –10, 58-62

11. *Suśrutasamhitā*, IV- 3,7,8,12,17.

12. *Carakasamhitā* VI - 5-44

13. *Aṣṭāṅgahṛdaya*, VI-12-84

14. *Naiṣadhīyacarita*, canto IV.116

15. *Śāstram Indiayil*, p.19

16. Dr. Raghavan Thirumulppad, *Āyurvedaparicayam*, p.30

17. *Op.cit.* p. 19.

18. Vāgbhaṭa, *Aṣṭāṅgasaṅgraha*, sūtrasthāna, 1/13-20

19. K.R Srikanthamurthy, Introduction to *Aṣṭāṅgasaṅgraha*, p X.

20. *Ibid.* uttarasthāna, 50/203-204

21. P.V Sharma, *Āyurveda – ka – Vaijñānik itihās*, p.179

22. Niścalakara, *Ratnaprabhā*, 1/65-68

23. *Jejjaṭa Nirantarapadavyākhyā*, cikitsāsthāna, 3/197

24. *iti śrī vaidyapatisimhaguptasūnu śrīmat Vāgbhaṭa viracite Aṣṭāṅgahrdayasamhitāyām*

25. *nāmnā khadiravaṭikā kathiteyam simhaguptena soḍhalasamgraha* – gadanigraha, Part I, p.232

26. P.V Sharma, *Vāgbhaṭavivecana*, p.377

27. Introductory verse, *Tantrayuktivicāra* - Ed. E.Muthuswamy Govt. of Kerala publication.

28. P.V Sharma, *Vāgbhaṭavivecana*, p.p.345-348

29. K.R Srikantha Murthy, Introduction to *Aṣṭāṅgasaṅgraha*, p.XII

30. P.V Sharma, *Vāgbhaṭavivecana*, p.348

31. Jejjaṭa, *Nirantarapadavyākhyā*, Cikitsāsthāna, P.V. Sharma, *Vāgbhaṭavivecana*, p.375

32. K.R. Srikanthamurthy. *Aṣṭāṅgasaṅgraha* (Ed) introduction, p.XIV

33. P.V Sharma, *Aṣṭāṅganighaṇṭu* (Ed.) Colophon in MSS No.3 *śrīmadvāgbhaṭācāryaviracitāyāmaṣṭāṅgahrdaya samhitāyam Aṣṭāṅganighaṇṭuḥ samāptaḥ*

34. Hemaraja sharma, *Introduction to Kāśyapasamhitā*

35. P.V sharma, *Aṣṭāṅganighaṇṭu*. Introduction, p.XIX

36. *Sūnunā simhaguptasya rasaratnasamuccayaḥ Rasaratnasamuccaya*, chapter 1/8 (Ed.) Ambikadatta sastry. Chaukhamba Amarabharati, varanasi 1988

37. P.V Sharma, *Āyurveda –ka – vaijñānik itihās*, p.482

38. K.R Srikanthamurthy, *Aṣṭāṅgasaṅgraha* (Ed.) introduction, p.XVI

39. P.V Sharma, *Vāgbhaṭavivecana*, p.p 77-79

40. Vāgbhaṭa, *Aṣṭāṅgahrdaya*, Uttarasthāna, 40/80

41. K.R. Srikanthamurthy, *Aṣṭāṅgasaṅgraha* introduction, p.XVII

42. *Aṣṭāṅgasaṅgraha*, Uttarasthāna, 40/85-88

43. *Mādhavanidāna*, concluding verse

44. A.B. Keith, *A history of sanskrit literature*, p.32.

45. *Śārṅgadharasamhitā*, I – 1

46. K. Raghvan Thirumulppad, Medical science, *Technical literature in Sanskrit*, p.65

47. *Ibid*

48. *Bhāvaprakāśasamhitā*, I-1

49. *Kāśyapasamhitā*, kalpasthāna, 12/6.

50. *Aṣṭāṅgahṛdaya*, 6/40 –88.

Chapter 5

AṢṬĀṄGAHṚDAYA: THEORY AND PRACTICE

Aṣṭāṅgahṛdaya is one of the authoritative treatises on Āyurveda. It has attracted the attention of medical men not only in this country but also of neighboring countries such as Arabia, Persia, Tibet, Germany and Srilanka.[1] Its popularity is substantiated by a large number of commentaries by Indian scholars and appreciation by scholars of many other countries. With its beauty and brevity of poetical composition, sequential arrangement of topics and clear description of precepts and practices of Āyurveda, it has earned its rightful place as one among the *'Bṛhat-trayī'- three great treatises* of Āyurveda. Kerala physicians follow *Aṣṭāṅgahṛdaya* for theory and practice. Hence a detailed study is attempted here.

Aṣṭāṅgahṛdaya in General

Aṣṭāṅgahṛdaya contains six *sthānas* (sections) each *sthāna* consisting of varying number of *adhyāyas* (chapters); the total number of chapters being 120. The text is composed entirely in poetry that can be easily learnt by heart. The *sthānas* (sections) and their important contents are:-

1. *Sūtrasthāna* – The first section has 30 chapters dealing with basic doctrines of Āyurveda, principles of health, prevention of diseases, properties of articles of diet and drugs, humoral physiology and pathology different kinds of diseases and methods of treatment.

2. *Śarīrasthāna* – This section has 6 chapters dealing with embryology, anatomy, physiology, physiognomy, physical and psychological constitutions, auspicious and inauspicious dreams and omens, signs of bad prognosis and of oncoming death.

3. *Nidānasthāna* – This section has 16 chapters describing the causes, premonitory symptoms, characteristic features and pathogenesis, of some important diseases coming within the realm of *kāyacikitsā* (treatment of body)

4. *Cikitsāsthāna* – This section has 22 chapters elaborating the methods of treatment of all major organic diseases including efficacious medicinal recipes, diet and care of the patient.

5. *Kalpasiddhisthāna* – This section has 6 chapters dealing with preparation of recipes, administration of purificatory therapies and management of complications; and principles of pharmacy.

6. *Uttarasthāna* – The sixth and the last section is devoted to the remaining seven branches of Āyurveda. It has 40 chapters in total; divided as follows, viz. 3 for *bālacikitsā* (Peadiatrics), 4 for *grahacikitsā* (Demonology/Psychiatry), 17 for *ūrdhvāṅgacikitsā* (diseases of organs in the head.) subdivided again 9 for *netracikitsā* (Ophthalmology), 2 for *karṇacikitsā* (Otology), 2 for *nāsācikitsā* (Rhinology), 2 for *mukhacikitsā* (mouth, teeth and throat), and 2 for *śiroroga* (diseases of the head). *śalyacikitsā* (Surgery) has 10 chapters; *daṃṣṭra* (Toxicology) has 4; *jarācikitsā* (*rasāyana*, Rejuvenation therapy, Geriatrics) and *vṛṣa* or *vājīkaraṇa* (Virilification therapy, Aphrodiasiacs) have one chapter each.

Author – His Life and Identity

Like other Sanskrit scholars the author of *Aṣṭāṅgahṛdaya* has not furnished either his name or any other information about himself anywhere in the text. Hence many of the present scholars both India and western have been, consistently attempting to identify this author but so far no conclusion has been arrived at. All the views are 'the most feasible assumptions only'. The following internal and external evidences form the basics for identification.

1. In the concluding verses of the text, the author states:

   "By churning the great ocean of the eight branches of medicinal science, a great store of nector – the *Aṣṭāṅgasaṅgraha* (name of a treatise) was obtained. From that store, this treatise (*Aṣṭāṅgahṛdaya*) which is more useful, has arisen separately for satisfying the less studious".[2]

By studying this, the person will be able to understand the Saṅgraha (*Aṣṭāṅgasaṅgraha*).[3]

2. The author of *Aṣṭāṅgasaṅgraha*, has furnished the following information about himself and his work in the concluding verses of that treatise:

"There was a great physician by name Vāgbhaṭa, who was my grandfather, I bear his name; from him was born Simhagupta and I am from him (Simhagupta); I was born in the Sindhu country. Having learnt the science from Avalokita, my preceptor and much more from my father and after studying a large number of texts on this science, this treatise (*Aṣṭāṅgasaṅgraha*) has been written, suitably classified (arranged into sections, chapters etc.) [4]

Elsewhere he states that it has been prepared in such a manner as is suitable to the age.[5]

3. In some manuscripts of *Aṣṭāṅgahṛdaya* there is a colophon at the end of *nidāna* and *uttarasthānas* which reads as:

"Thus ends the *nidānasthāna* in *Aṣṭāṅgahṛdaya samhitā* written by Śrīmad Vāgbhaṭa, son of Śrī Vaidyapati Simhagupta".

But the absence of such a colophon at other places and in some other manuscripts, and the use of honorific term '*śrīmad*' as a prefix to the author's name have prompted the present day scholars to doubt the authenticity of the colophon.

4. Commentators on other Āyurveda treatises have quoted verses of *Aṣṭāṅgasaṅgraha* and of *Aṣṭāṅgahṛdaya* with the description as 'from *vṛddha* Vāgbhaṭa' and 'from *laghu/svalpa* Vāgbhaṭa respectively.

Based on these points, it is now generally agreed that the author of *Aṣṭāṅgahṛdaya* is also Vāgbhaṭa. Whether *Aṣṭāṅgahṛdaya* and *Aṣṭāṅgasaṅgraha* were written by one and the same person — Vāgbhaṭa, son of Simhagupta or whether the authors are different persons of the same name has already been discussed in the previous sections of the study.

Further a comparison of *Aṣṭāṅgasaṅgraha* and *Aṣṭāṅgahṛdaya* is given as follows:

Aṣṭāṅgasaṅgraha	*Aṣṭāṅgahṛdaya*
Nature of composition	
a) Archaic style containing both prose & poetry, with difficult words, long sentences.	New style containing only verses, easily understandable
b) Contains detailed description of religious practices, social customs and believes etc.	Brief narration of religious matters etc.
Number of Verses.	
9241 (prose passages and verses together)	7120 (only verses)

	Aṣṭāṅgasaṅgraha	*Aṣṭāṅgahṛdaya*
Number of sthānas (sections)	6	6
Number of *adhyayas* (chapters)		
a. *sūtrasthāna*	40	30
b. *śarīrasthāna*	12	6
c. *nidānasthāna*	16	16
d. *cikitsāsthāna*	24	22
e. *kalpasiddhisthāna*	8	6
f. *uttarasthāna*	50	40
	150	120

Topic wise break — up in *uttarasthāna*

Topic	Number of Adhyāyas	
a) *bālacikitsā*	5	3
b) *grahacikitsā*	5	4
c) *ūrdhvāṅgacikitsā* :		
i) *netrarogacikitsā*	10	9
ii) *karṇacikitsā*	2	2
iii) *nāsāroga*	2	2
iv) *mukharoga*	2	2
v) *śiroroga*	2	2

d) *śalyacikitsā*	11	10
e) *damṣṭrā (viṣa) cikitsā*	9	4
f) *jarācikitsā (rasāyana)*	1	1
g) *vṛṣa (vājīkaraṇa)*	1	1
	50	40

In this connection, attention may be drawn to the interesting argument put forward by Dr. K.R Srikantha Murthy in his introduction to *Aṣṭāṅgahṛdaya* about the order of sequence of these texts, *Aṣṭāṅgahṛdaya* and *Aṣṭāṅgasaṅgraha*. Dr. K.R Srikantha Murthy observes thus:

1. "There are two divergent opinions regarding the order of sequence of these texts. Viz. (1) all Indian scholars consider that *Aṣṭāṅgasaṅgraha* is the earlier text and *Aṣṭāṅgahṛdaya*, the later. (2) European scholars consider the *Aṣṭāṅgahṛdaya* is earlier, next an intermediary text and *Aṣṭāṅgasamgraha* is the last. Points in support of this view are — *Aṣṭāṅgahṛdaya* was popular in neighboring countries and has been translated into Arabian and Tibetan languages very early but not *Aṣṭāṅgasamgraha*; there are more number of commentaries on *Aṣṭāṅgahṛdaya* and it is included among the *bṛhattrayī*- great triad of Āyurveda literature, where as *Aṣṭāṅgasaṅgraha* does not have these Privileges. With the above two conflicting views, it is better to keep this topic open for some more time anticipating further research [6]

Date of Vāgbhaṭa

The date of Vāgbhaṭa the author of *Aṣṭāṅgahṛdaya* and *Aṣṭāṅgasaṅgraha* can be determined from the following evidences.

1. Many recipes found in the *Bower MSS* are also found in *Aṣṭāṅgahṛdaya*. The *Bower MSS* is assigned to IV century AD and Vāgbhaṭa might have borrowed the recipes from it.

2. In *Aṣṭāṅgahṛdaya*, Vāgbhaṭa has quoted verses from that portion of *Carakasamhitā* which has been supplemented by Dṛḍhabala, who belongs to about 500 AD. This is the upper limit of the date of the Vāgbhaṭa.

3. *Bṛhatsaṃhitā* of Varāhamihira has a verse which very closely resembles the verse of *Aṣṭāṅgahṛdaya* and most probably taken from it. Varāhamihira lived in between 505 and 580 AD. This date is taken as the lower limit for the date of Vāgbhaṭa.

4. Itsing, the Chinese traveller in his travel records (671-695 AD), states that 'lately a person collected all the eight branches of medicine, neither to separate and made them into, one bundle.[7] This in all probability refers to Vāgbhaṭa.

5. The religious, social and economic conditions described in *Aṣṭāṅgasaṅgraha* and *Aṣṭāṅgahṛdaya* pertain to the early phase of Gupta era of Indian history. (5th – 7th AD)

6. *Aṣṭāṅgahṛdaya* has been translated into Arabic by the name *Astankar* during the reign of Khalif Harun-al- Rashid (773 – 808 AD)[8]

From the above evidences it is pertinent to infer his date as between 550-600 AD.

A detailed account of *Aṣṭāṅgahṛdaya* is attempted in the next section.

Aṣṭāṅgahṛdaya – a textual analysis

It is already mentioned that the text contains six sections called six *sthānas* namely *sūtra, śarīra, nidāna, cikitsā, kalpa* and *uttara* respectively.

Sūtrasthāna

Sūtrasthāna consists of 1631 *kārikas* (verses) in all. The verses are distributed among thirty chapters as following:

Numbers & Name of adhyaya (chapters)		Number of Verses
1.	*āyuṣkāmīya* (Longevity)	49
2.	*Dinacaryā* (Daily regimen)	49
3.	*ṛtucaryā* (Seasonal regimen)	58

Numbers & Name of adhyaya (chapters)	Number of Verses
4. *Rogānulpādanīya* (Prevention of Diseases)	35
5. *Dravadravyavijñānīya* (Knowledge of liquid materials)	90
6. *Annasvarūpavijñānīya* (Nature of food materials)	173
7. *Annarakṣādhyāya* (Protection of foods)	77
8. *Mātrāśitiya* (Partaking proper quantity of food)	55
9. *Dravyādivijñānīya* (Knowledge of substances etc)	29
10. *Rasabhedīya* (Classification of tastes)	44
11. *Doṣādivijñānīya* (Knowledge of doṣas etc)	46
12. *Doṣabhedīya* (Classification of doṣas)	79
13. *Doṣāpakramanīya* (Treatment of the doṣas)	41
14. *Dvividhopakramaṇīya* (Two kinds of treatment)	37
15. *śodhanādigaṇasaṅgraha* (Groups of drugs for purificatory therapies etc)	47
16. *snehavidhi* (Oleation therapy)	46
17. *svedavidhi* (Sedation therapy)	30
18. *vamanavirecanavidhi* (Emesis and purgation therapies)	59

Numbers & Name of adhyaya (chapters)	Number of Verses
19. *vastividhi* (Enema therapy)	87
20. *nasyavidhi* (Nasal medication)	57
21. *dhūmapānavidhi* (Inhalation of Smoke)	23
22. *gaṇḍūṣadividhi* (Mouth gargles and other therapies)	35
23. *aścotana – añjanavidhi* (Eye drops, eye-salves therapy)	31
24. *tarpaṇa puṭapākavidhi* (Satiating the eye and other therapies)	23
25. *yantravidhi* (Usage of blunt instruments and appliances)	43
26. *śastravidhi* (Usage of sharp instruments)	55
27. *Sirāvyādhavidhi* (procedure of Venesection)	53
28. *śalyāharaṇavidhi* (Removal of foreign bodies)	48
29. *śastrakarmavidhi* (Procedure of surgical operation)	79
30. *kṣārāgnikarmavidhi* (Procedure of cauterisation)	53

The first section of the *Aṣṭāṅgahṛdaya* named *sūtrasthāna* (section on general principles) begins with *ayuṣkāmīya adhyāya* (desire for long life). This chapter begins with the salutation to *Apūrvavaidya* as follows.

Rāgādirogān satatānuṣaktān

Aśeṣakāyaprasṛtānaśeṣān /

Autsukyamoho'ratitān jaghāna

Yo'pūrvavaidyāya namo'stu tasmai. // [9]

Obeisances be, to that Unique/rare physician who has destroyed, without any residue (all) the diseases like rāga (passion/desire) etc. which are constantly associated (innate/inherent) with and spread all over the body, giving rise to *autsukya* (anxiety), *moha* (delution) and *arati* (restlessness).

It deserves special mention that Vāgbhaṭa begins his work with the salutation to *Apūrvavaidya* instead of any *iṣṭadevatā* (god) because of the influence of Buddhism.

Then origin of Āyurveda is described as follows:

Brahmā smṛtvāyuṣo vedam prajāpatimajigrahat /

So'śvinau tau sahasrākṣam so'triputrādikānmunīn /

Te'gniveśādikāmste tu pṛthak tantrāṇi tenire // [10]

Brahman, remembering Āyurveda (the science of life) taught it to Prajāpati, he (Prajāpati) in turn taught it to Aśvin twins, they taught it to Sahasrākṣa (Indra) he taught to it Atris son (Ātreya punarvasu or Kṛṣṇa Ātreya) and other sages, they taught it to Agniveśa and others and they (Agniveśa and other disciples) composed treatises each one separately.

It can be seen that the above is a brief narration of origin of Āyurveda according to *Carakasamhitā*. [11]

The composition of *Aṣṭāṅgahṛdaya* is described in the next portion thus:

Tebhyo'tiviprakīrṇebhyaḥ prāyaḥ sārataroccayaḥ /

Kriyate'ṣṭāṅgahṛdayam nātisamkṣepavistaram // [12]

From those treatises which are very elaborate (hence difficult to study), only the essence has been collected and this treatise – *Aṣṭāṅgahṛdaya* – prepared which is neither too succinct nor too elaborate.

Eight branches of Āyurveda (*Aṣṭāṅgāyurveda*) are mentioned in the next verse.

Kāyabālagrahordhvāṅgaśalyadamṣṭrājarāvṛṣān /

aṣṭāvaṅgāni tasyāhuścikitsā yeṣu samśritā // [13]

kāya, bāla, graha, ūrdhvāṅga, śalya, damṣṭrā, jarā and *vṛṣa* are the eight branches (of Āyurveda) in which treatment (of diseases) is embodied.

These eight branches are respectively Inner medicine, pediatrics, psychiatry, ophthalmology, surgery, toxicology, geriatrics and aphrodisiacs in modern medicine respectively.

Tridoṣas (Three humours) responsible for the maintenance of the health are descrbied thus:

> *Vāyuḥ pittam kaphaśceti trayo doṣāḥ samāsataḥ /*
>
> *Vikṛtāvikṛtā deham ghnanti te vardhyanti ca //* [14]

Vāyu (*vāta*), *pitta* and *kapha* are three *doṣas*, in brief they destroy and support (sustain, maintain) the body when they are abnormal and normal respectively.

The *doṣas* are material substances present in the body and always they have their own definite *pramāṇa* (Quantity), *guṇa* (Quality) and *Karma* (functions). When they are normal (*avikṛta*) they attend to different functions of the body and so maintain it. But they have the tendency to become abnormal (*vikṛta*) undergoing increase (*vṛddhi*) or decrease (*kṣaya*) in their quantity, one or more of their qualities and functions. When they become abnormal, they vitiate their places of dwelling. The *dhātus* (tissues) because of this tendency of vitiation, they are called as dosas or vitiators.

Roga (disease) is defined as *doṣavaiṣamyam* and health is as *doṣasāmya* thus:

> *rogastu doṣavaiṣamyam*
>
> *doṣasāmyamarogatā //* [15]

Roga (disease) is (the effect of) disequilibrium of the *doṣas* while health is (the result of) the equilibrium of the *doṣas*.

Rogas (diseases) are classified as two as follows:

> *Nijāgantuvibhāgena tatra rogā dvidhāsmṛtaḥ /* [16]

Roga (disease) is said to be of two kinds, *nija* (organic, arising from the body itself) and *āgantu* (traumatic, arising from external causes)

It is interesting here to note that modern medicine also classifies diseases into two,[17] somewhat similar to the above division; life style diseases and infectious diseases.

Rogī – rogaparīkṣā (examination of the patient) is described as follows:

Darśanasparśanapraśnaiḥ parīkṣeta ca roginam [18]

The *rogin* (patient) should be examined by *darśana* (inspection) *sparśana* (palpation) and *praśna* (interrogation)

The identification of a disease (*roga*) is described as follows:

rogam nidānaprāgrūpalakṣaṇopaśayāptibhiḥ // [19]

roga (disease) should examined by its *nidāna* (causes), *prāgrūpa* (premonitory symptoms), *lakṣaṇa* (specific signs and symptoms) *upāśaya* (diagnostic tests) and *āpti* (*samprāpti*, pathogenesis)

Āyurveda gives more emphasis to 'go with the nature', believing in the maxim that prevention is better than cure. There is a separate chapter for daily regimen (*dinacaryādhyāya*) allotted for this purpose. In *ṛtucaryādhyāya* (Seasonal regimen) six *ṛtus* are mentioned.

Māsaidvisamkhairmāghādyaiḥ kramāt ṣaṭ ṛtavaḥ smṛtāḥ /

śiśiro 'tha vasantaśca grīṣmo varṣaśaraddhimāḥ // [20]

With every two *māsa* (months) commencing with *māgha*, are the six *ṛtus* (seasons) *śiśira, vasanta, grīṣma, varṣa* and *hima* (*hemanta*)

From the description of six *ṛtus* here one can definitely infer that the author of *Aṣṭāṅgahṛdaya* seems to be a non - Keralite because in Kerala only four seasons are available namely *varṣa, śarat, vasanta, grīṣma*.

As indicated earlier Āyurveda gives emphasis to the prevention of diseases than cure. There is a separate chapter named *rogānulpādanīya* (prevention of disease) devoted for this purpose. In this chapter the essence of Āyurveda is given as follows:

nityam hitāhāravihārasevī

samīkṣyakārī viṣayeṣvasaktaḥ /

dātā samaḥ satyaparaḥ kṣamāvān

āptopasevī ca bhavatyarogaḥ // [21]

One, who indulges daily in healthy foods and activities, who discriminates (the good and bad of everything and then acts wisely), who is not attached (too much) to the object of senses, who develops the habit of charity, of considering all as equal (requiring kindness), of truthfulness, of pardoning and keeping company of good persons only, becomes free from all diseases.

It is interesting to see that the first portion of this verse gives importance to physical activities and second portion to mental activities respectively.

In the *dravadravyavijñānīya* chapter knowledge of liquid materials is described. The qualities of coconut water is sighted here by way of illustration

Nāḷikerodakam snigdham svādu vṛṣyam himam laghu /

Tṛṣṇāpittānilaharam dīpanam vastiśodhanam // [22]

Nāḷikerodaka (coconut water) is unctuous, sweet, aphrodisiac, coolant, easily diagestable, relieves thirst, (aggravation of) *pitta* and *anila* (*vāta*), increases hunger and cleanses the Urinary bladder,

In *annasamrakṣaṇīya* chapter sleeping during day time is prohibited. It may causes the following difficulties as follows:

akālaśayanānmohajvarastaimityapīnasāḥ /

śirorukkāsaśophahṛllasasrotorodhāgnimandatāḥ // [23]

Sleeping at improper time causes delusion, fever, lassitude, nasal catarch, headache, dropsy, oppression in the chest (nausea), obstruction of the tissue pores and weakness of digestive function.

In *doṣabhedīya* chapter the importance of practice (*abhyāsa*) is clearly emphasised for successful treatment thus:

Abhyāsātprāpyate dṛṣṭiḥ karmasiddhiprakāśinī /

Ratnādisadasajjñānam na śāstrādeva jāyate // [24]

Knowledge of successful treatment is obtained from constant practice just as knowledge of (determining) good or bad gems etc is not obtained only from (knowing) the science.

The qualities of meet food are mentioned in *dvividhopakramaṇīya* chapter.

na hi māmsasamam kiñcidanyaddehabṛhatvakṛt /

māmsādamāmsam māmsena sambhṛtatvādviśeṣataḥ // [25]

There is nothing other than meat to stouten the body, especially so the is the case of the meat of carnivorous animals, as they feed on meat itself.

This verse indicates that at the time of Vāgbhaṭa, no taboo was attached to meat eating.

Sūtrasthāna concludes with the declaration that this section is the most important one thus:

Samāpyate sthānamidam hṛdayasya rahasyavat /

Atrārthāḥ sūtritāḥ sūksmāḥ pratanyante hi sarvataḥ // [26]

Thus will be concluded, this section of *Aṣṭāṅgahṛdaya* which is full of secrets, for in it are codified all the chief doctrines which are described in detail everywhere. (In the entire treatise).

The idea behind this concluding verse is that this section is an epitome of Āyurveda and without a study of *sūtrasthāna* in the beginning it will be very difficult to understand the contents of the other sections of the treatise, because the doctrines are mentioned in this section and only other details are found in other sections.

Śarīrasthāna

Śarīrasthāna (anatomy & physiology), the second section of *Aṣṭāṅgahṛdaya* consists of 561 verses. These verses are distributed among 6 chapters.

Sl. No	Number and Name of *adhyāya* (chapter)	Number of verses
1.	*garbhāvakrāntiśarīra* (Embryology)	100
2.	*garbhavyāpadśarīra* (Disorders of Pregnancy)	62
3.	*aṅgavibhāgaśarīram* (Different parts of the body)	120
4.	*marmavibhāgaśarīra* (Classification of vital spots)	74
5.	*vikṛtivisnyānīya* (Knowledge of bad prognostics)	131
6.	*dūtavijñānīya* (Knowledge about the messenger)	74
	Total	561

This section begins with the chapter on *garbhāvakrānti* (Embryology). It mentions the ideal time for the marriage and a warning against the child marriage.

pūrṇaṣoḍaśavarṣā strī pūrṇa vimśena saṅgatā

śuddhe garbhāśaye mārge rakte śukḷe'nile hṛdi /

vīryavantam sutam sūte tayonnyūnabdayoḥ punaḥ

rogyālpāyuradhānyo vā garbho bhavati naiva vā // [27]

The woman who has completed sixteen years of age, when mate with a man who has completed twenty years, gives birth to a valiant son, as the uterus, the channels, the blood (menstrual), semen, *anila* (*vata*) and *hṛdaya* (the wind, in this context) are pure (unvitiated). On the other hand, if the age is less, the offspring will be either sick, of short life, of inauspicious nature or there may be no formation of fetus at all.

The qualities of five primary elements (*pañcabhūta*) are given and how they take part in the formation of physical body are also explained thus:

śabdaḥ sparśaśca rūpam ca raso gandhaḥ kramād guṇāḥ /

khānilāgnibhuvāmekaguṇavṛdhyanvayāḥ pare

tatra khāt khāni dehe'smin śrotram śabdo viviktatā I

vātātsparśatvagucchvāsa vahnerdṛgrūpapaktayaḥ

āpyā jihvārasakledā ghrāṇagandhāsthi pārthivam // [28]

śabda (sound), *sparśa* (touch), *rūpa* (form), *rasa* (taste) and *gandha* (smell) are the qualities of *kham* (*ākāśa*), *anila* (*vāyu*), *agni* (*tejas*), *ambu* (*ap*) and *bhū* (*pṛthvī*) respectively. Progressive increase one more quality is found in each succeeding element (*bhūta*). In this human body, from *pṛthvībhūta* are (produced) the orifices (tubes, channels, pores), the ears (organs of sound perception), the sound (voice, sound of the heart, lungs, intestine etc) and empty spaces (*ākāśa*). From *vāyubhūta* are (produced) the touch, the skin (organ of touch perception) and respiration. From *agnibhūta* are (produced) the eyes (organs of perception of light), vision and digestion. From *apbhūta* are (produced) the tongue (organ of taste perception), taste, fluids and moisture. From *pṛthvībhūta* are (produced) the nose (organ of perception of smell), the smell and the bones.

At the end of this section the qualities required for a patient are given as follows:

Maṅgalācārasampannaḥ parivārāstathāturaḥ

śraddhadhāno'nukūlaśca prabhūtadravyasaṅgrahaḥ /

satvalakṣaṇasamyogo bhaktirvaidyadvijātiṣu

cikitsāyāmanirvedastadārogyasya lakṣaṇam // [29]

The attendants endowed with good conduct, having faith, helpful with plenty of money, obedient to the physician and the twice born (*brāhmaṇa*) enthusiastic about the treatment are the factors of health (regaining health).

Nidānasthāna

Nidānasthāna (diagnosis of diseases), the third section of *Aṣṭāṅgahṛdaya* consists of 787 verses. The verses are distributed among 16 chapters as followings:

Sl.No.	Number & name of *adhyāya*	Number of verses
1.	*sarvaroganidānam* (diagnosis of disease in general)	24
2.	*jvarānidānam* (diagnosis of fever)	79
3.	*raktapitta-kāsanidānam* (diagnosis of bleeding diseases and cough)	38
4.	*śvāsa-hidhmānidānam* (diagnosis of dyspnoea and hiccup)	31
5.	*Rājayakṣmādinidānam* (diagnosis of pulmonary tuberculosis)	57
6.	*Madātyayanidānam* (diagnosis of alcoholic intoxication)	41
7.	*arśasnidānam* (diagnosis of haemorrhoids)	59
8.	*atisāra-grahaṇīnidānam* (diagnosis of diarrhoea and duodenal disorders)	30
9.	*Mūtraghātanidānam* (diagnosis of retention of urine)	40
10.	*pramehanidānam* (diagnosis of diabetes)	41
11.	*vidradhi-vṛddhi-gulmanidānam* (diagnosis of abscess, enlargement of the scrotum and abdominal tumour)	63

12.	*udaranidānam* (diagnosis of enlargement of the abdomen)	46
13.	*pāṇḍuroga-śopha-visarpanidānam* (diagnosis of anaemia, drospy and herpes)	67
14.	*kuṣṭha-śvitra-kṛminidānam* (diagnosis of leprosy, leucoderma, and parasites)	56
15.	*vātavyādhinidānam* (diagnosis of the nervous system)	57
16.	*vataśoṇitanidānam* (daignosis of gout)	58

This section begins with the indication of 11 synonyms to the term disease thus:

rogaḥ pāpma jvara vyādhirvikāro duhkhāmāmayaḥ /

yakṣmātaṅkagadabādhāḥ śabdāḥ paryāyavācakaḥ // [30]

roga, pāpma, jvara, vyādhi, vikāra, duḥkha, āmaya, yakṣmā, ātaṅka, gada and ābādha — these terms are synonyms.

Prof. K. R Srikantha Murthy points out that each of these terms indicates a certain aspect of the disease. The disease is called *roga* because it gives rise to pain, it is *pāpma* because it is born from sinful acts, *jvara* because it torments, *vyādhi* for it brings in different kinds of abnormalities, *duḥkha*, as it various kinds of unhappiness, *āmaya* because it is caused by *āma* (undigested, improperly processed metabolites), *yakṣmā* as it is a group of diseases (symptom complex, syndrome), *ātaṅka* for it makes life miserable, *gada* because it is produced by multiple causes, *ābādha* for it produces constant discomfort (to the body, mind or sense organs). [31]

Five means of diagnosis required for the diagnosis of a diseases is given as follows:

(The five means of diagnosis-*nidāna* (cause). *Pūrvarūpa* (premonitory symptoms), *rūpa* (signs and symptoms) characteristic of the diseases) *upaśaya* (diagnostic test) and *samprāpti* (mode of manifestation of the diseases) are five means of obtaining fill knowledge (diagnosis) of diseases). [32]

It is interesting to note that in *pramehanidāna* chapter among the other causes for Diabetes, habit of always sitting at a place and sleeping without adopting its proper procedure (sleeping during day time) are also included. *ekasthānāsanaratiḥ śayanam vidhivarjitam.*[33] Now a days modern medicine also considers Diabetes as a life style disease. This section concludes with the causes of different type of *vāta* (gout) diseases.

Cikitsāsthāna

Cikitsāsthāna (section on therapeutics) of *Aṣṭāṅgahṛdaya* consists of 1976 verses. These verses are distributed among 22 chapter as follows.

Sl.No	Number & Name of *adhyaya*	Number of verses
1.	*jvarācikitsā* (treatment of fevers)	177
2.	*raktapittacikitsā* (treatment of bleeding diseases	50
3.	*kāsacikitsā* (treatment of cough)	180
4.	*śvāsa-hidhmā cikitsita* (treatment of dyspnoea and hiccup)	59
5.	*Rājayakṣmādicikitsā* (treatment of pulmonary tuberculosis etc)	83
6.	*charddi – hṛdroga – tṛṣṇā cikitsā* (treatment of vomitting, heart diseases and thirst)	84
7.	*madātyayacikitsā* (treatment of alcoholic intoxination)	115
8.	*arśascikitsā* (treatment of haemorrhoids)	164
9.	*atisāracikitsā* (treatment of diarrhoea)	124

10.	*grahaṇidosacikitsā* (treatment of duodenal disorder)	93
11.	*mūtrāghātacikitsā* (treatment of retention of urine)	63
12.	*pramehacikitsā* (treatment of diabetes)	44
13.	*vidradhi-vṛddhicikitsā* (treatment of abscess, enlargement of the scrotum)	52
14.	*gulmacikitsā* (treatment of abdominal tumour)	129
15.	*udaracikitsitā* (treatment of enlargement of the abdomen)	132
16.	*pāṇḍurogacikitsā* (treatment of anaemia)	57
17.	*śvayathu (śopha)cikitsā* (treatment of dropsy)	42
18.	*visarpacikitsā* (treatment of herps)	38
19.	*kuṣṭhacikitsā* (treatment of leprosy)	98
20.	*śvitrakṛmicikitsā* (treatment of leucoderma and parasites)	35
21.	*Vātavyādhicikitsā* (treatment of the diseases of the nervous system)	83
22.	*Vātaśoṇitacikitsā* (treatment of gout)	74

After describing various treatment for all the diseases mentioned above Vāgbhaṭa concludes this section thus:

Yathānidānam nirdiṣṭamiti samyak cikitsitam

āyurvedaphalam sthānametatsadyortināśanāt /

cikitsitam hitam pathyam prāyaścittam bhiṣagjitam

bheṣajam śamanam śastam paryāyaiḥ smṛtamauṣadham // [34]

In this manner, the treatment of all the diseases described in the *nidānasthāna* are elaborated in this chapters which yields the benefit of Āyurveda and destroys the sufferings (of men). *Auṣadha* (treatments) is known by many synonyms such as *cikitsita, hita, pathya, prāyaścitta, bhiṣagjita, śamana and śasta*.

Kalpasiddhisthāna

Kalpasiddhisthāna (pharamaceutics & purificatory recipes) consists of 305 verse. These verses

Sl.No.	Number & Name of Adhyaya	Number of verses
1.	*vamanakalpa* (Emetic recipes)	47
2.	*virecanakalpa* (Purgative recipes)	62
3.	*vamanavirecanavyāpatsiddhi* (Management of complications of Emesis and purgation therapies)	39
4.	*vastikalpa* (Enema recipes)	73
5.	*vastivyāpatsiddhi* (Management of complications of enema therapy)	54
6.	*dravyakalpa* (Pharmaceutics)	30

The keen power of observation of the author can be gathered from the description of medicinal herbs.:

Himavadvindhyaśailābhyām prāyo vyāptā vasundharā

saumyam pathyam ca tatrādyamāgneyam vaindhyamauṣadham // [35]

The herbs are found in the Himavat and Vindhya mountains generally, of them, those from the first (Himavat) are saumya (cold, coolent, mild in action) and good for health; whereas those from Vindhya mountains are *āgneya* (hot, firy, strong in action)

Uttarasthāna

Uttarasthāna is the last section of *Aṣṭāṅgahṛdaya*. It consists of 2234 verses. These are distributed among 40 chapters as follows.

Sl.No.	Number & Name of *adhyāya*	Number of verses
1.	*bālopacāraṇīya* (Care of the new born baby)	49
2.	*bālāmayapratiṣedha* (Treatment of diseases if children)	78
3.	*bālagrahapratiṣedha* (Treatment of evil spirits)	60
4.	*bhūtavijñānīya* (Knowledge of Demons)	44
5.	*bhūtapratiṣedha* (Treatment of Demons)	53
6.	*unmādapratiṣedha* (Treatment of insanity)	60
7.	*apasmārapratiṣedha* (Treatment of epilepsy)	37
8.	*vartmarogavijñānīya* (Knowledge of diseases of eyelids)	27
9.	*vartmarogaprtiṣedha* (Treatment of diseases of eyelids)	41
10.	*sandhisitasitārogavijñānīya* (Knowledge of diseases of fornices, sclera and cornea)	31

11.	*sandhisitāsitarogapratiṣedha* (Treatment of diseases of fornices, sclera and cornea)	58
12.	*dṛṣṭirogavijñānīya* (Knowledge of diseases of vision)	33
13.	*timirapratiṣedha* (Treatment of blindness)	100
14.	*liṅganāśapratiṣedha* (Treatment of blindness)	32
15.	*sarvākṣirogavijñānīya* (Knowledge of diseases of the whole eye)	24
16.	*sarvākṣirogapratiṣedha* (Treatment of diseases of the whole body)	67
17.	*karṇarogavijñānīya* (Knowledge of diseases of the ear)	26
18.	*karṇarogapratiṣedha* (Treatment of diseases of the ear)	66
19.	*nāsārogavijñānīya* (Knowledge of diseases of the nose)	27
20.	*nāsārogapratiṣedha* (Treatment of disease of the nose)	25
21.	*mukharogavijñānīya* (Knowledge of disease of the mouth)	69
22.	*mukharogapratiṣedha* (Treatment of disease of the mouth)	111
23.	*śirorogavijñānīya* (Knowledge of diseases of the head)	32
24.	*śirorogapratiṣedha* (Treatment of disease of the head)	59

25.	*Vraṇapratiṣedha* (Treatment of ulcers)	67
26.	*Sadyovraṇapratiṣedha* (Treatment of traumatic wounds)	58
27.	*Bhaṅgapratiṣedha* (Treatment of fractures)	41
28.	*bhagandarapratiṣedha* (Treatment of rectal fistula)	44
29.	*grandhi-arbuda-ślīpada-apacinadivijñānīya* (Knowledge of tumors, cancers, filariasis, scrofila and sinus ulcer)	31
30.	*granthyādipratiṣedha* (Treatment of tumours etc)	40
31.	*kṣudrarogavijñānīya* (Knowledge of minor diseases)	33
32.	*kṣudrarogapratiṣedha* (Treatment of minor diseases)	33
33.	*guhyarogavijñānīya* (Knowledge of diseases of genital organs)	52
34.	*guhyarogapratiṣedha* (Treatment of diseases of genital organs)	67
35.	*viṣapratiṣedha* (Treatment of poisoning)	70
36.	*sarpaviṣapratiṣedha* (Treatment of snake bite poison)	93
37.	*kīṭālūtādiviṣapratiṣedha* (Treatment of poison of insects, spiders etc)	86

38.	*mūṣika-alarkaviṣapratiṣedha* (Treatment of poison of mouse, rabbit, dog etc)	40
39.	*rasāyanavidhi* (Rejuvination therapy)	181
40.	*vājīkaraṇavidhi* (Virilification therapy)	89

Uttarasthāna, forms one third of the total number of chapters and is very comprehensive and practical. So it is very valuable to the students of Āyurveda like *sūtrasthāna*.

Apart from the other subjects the author give importance to *rasāyanavidhi* (Rejuvention therapy). Benefits of *rasāyanavidhi* are described as follows:

dīrghamāyuḥ smṛtim medhāmārogyam taruṇam vayaḥ

prabhāvarṇasvaraudārya dehendriyabalodayam /

vāksiddhim vṛṣatām kāntimavāpnoti rasāyanāt

lābhopāyo hi śastānām rasādīnām rasāyanam // [36]

Long life, (good) memory (great) intelligence (perfect) health, youthfulness, (bright) complexion and colour, bold (voice) and magnanimity increase of strength of the body and the sense organs perfection in speech, sexual prowess and brilliance are all obtained from *rasāyana* therapy. It is the best means of keeping the *rasa* and other *dhātus* in excellent condition.

After describing different types of *rasāyanavidhis*, Vāgbhaṭa insists that this therapy is complete only under the following conditions.

śāstranusāriṇī caryā cittajñaḥ pārśvavartinaḥ /

Buddhiraskhalitārtheṣu paripūrṇam rasāyanam // [37]

Rejuvenatory therapy is complete when indulgence in activities as ordained by the scriptures, understanding of the mind of the persons near by, and mind unwavering by the (effect of) objects (of sense organs) become possible.

At the concluding portion of the *Aṣṭāṅgahṛdaya*, Vāgbhaṭa describes the nature of the composition of the work thus:

iti tantragaṇairuktam tantradoṣavivarjitam

cikitsāśāstramakhilam vyāpārya paritasthitam /

vipulāmalavijñānamahāmunimatānugam

mahāsāgaragambhīrasamgrahārthopalakṣaṇam //

aṣṭāṅgavaidyakamahodadhimanthanena

yo 'ṣṭāṅgasaṅgrahamahāmṛtarāśirāptaḥ

tasmādanalpaphalamalpasamudyamānām

prītyarthametaduditam pṛthageva tantram // [38]

Following the techniques of the great sages who possessed unlimited and unvitiated knowledge arose the *Saṅgraha* (*Aṣṭāṅgasaṅgraha*) which is deep like the great Ocean. This text (*Aṣṭāṅgahṛdaya*) is an epitome. By churning the great Ocean of the eight branches of medical science a great store of - the *Aṣṭāṅgasaṅgraha* was obtained. From that *Aṣṭāṅgasaṅgraha* is born this text (*Aṣṭāṅgahṛdaya*) separately which is greatly beneficial for satisfying the less studious.

Vāgbhaṭa declares the merit of his work in comparable to Caraka and Suśruta thus:

Etatpaṭhan samgrahabodhasaktaḥ

svabhyastakarma bhiṣagaprakampyaḥ /

ākampayatyanyaviśālatantra

kṛtābhiyogān yadi tanna citram //

yadi carakamadhīte tad dhruvam suśrutādi

praṇigaditagadānām nāmamātre 'pi bāhyaḥ

atha carakavihīnaḥ prakiyāyāmakhinnaḥ

kimiva khalu karotu vyādhitānām varākaḥ // [39]

By studying this text, the physician will be able to understand the *Saṅgraha* (*Aṣṭāṅgasaṅgraha*), becomes well versed and dextrous in his professional work. What is strange if he makes other (physicians) who have studied still bigger texts tremble. He (physician) who reads only the *Caraka* (*samhitā*) is deprived of ever the names of the diseases which are described by *Suśruta* (*samhitā*) etc; and he who is devoid of (not studied) *Caraka* (*samhitā*) becomes inefficient in giving treatment. What good can such an unintelligent man do to the patient?

Even though *Aṣṭāṅgahṛdaya* got recognition nowadays, the concluding portion of the text makes it imperative for us, to assume that Vāgbhaṭa had not attained an authoritative status during his life time and that his works were not accepted as scriptures of Āyurveda. This can be observed from his own words thus

Abhiniveśavaśādabhiyujyate

Subhaṇite 'pi na yo dṛḍhamūḍhakaḥ /

Paṭhatu yatnaparaḥ puruṣāyuṣam

sa khalu vaidyakamādyamanirvidaḥ // [40]

He the stubborn fool, who filled with prejudice, does not appreciate a text even though it is well composed let him, study with all effort through out his life, the first medical text itself composed by Lord Brahmā.

And also

abhidhātṛvaśāt kimvā dravyaśaktirviśiṣyate ato /

mātsaramutsṛjya mādhyasthyamavalambyatām // [41]

Is there any special difference in the power (action of the drugs, if described by any specific person? Hence adopt the middle path (avoiding both extremes), casting away the jealousy (prejudice against *Aṣṭāṅgahṛdaya* and its author)

Further Vāgbhaṭa argues thus:

ṛṣipraṇīte prītiścet muktvā carakasuśrutau /

bhedādyāḥ kim na paṭhyante tasmād grāhyam subhāṣitam // [42]

(If there is love for the work of sages only then why don't people read the work of *Bheda* etc, keeping away the work of Caraka and Suśruta? So, any good word (text) should be accepted.)

Vāgbhaṭa concludes his text by wishing happiness to the whole world.

hṛdayamiva hṛdayametat

sarvāyurvedavāṅmayapayodheḥ /

kṛtvā yacchubhamāptam

subhamastu param tato jagataḥ // [43]

This *Hṛdaya (Aṣṭāṅgahṛdaya)* is like the heart (essence) of the entire ocean of literature of Āyurveda. From the good fortune that accrues from it, let the whole world attain happiness.

Important commentaries on *Aṣṭāṅgahṛdaya*

Aṣṭāṅgahṛdaya of Vāgbhaṭa possesses the highest number of commentaries in conformity with its popularity. Though about thirty commentaries are known most of them are either lost, available partly or remaining in manuscript form. It is already mentioned that *Aṣṭāṅgahṛdaya* is accepted as an authentic text by Kerala physicians. So it has a large number of commentaries in Sanskrit and Malayalam by Keralite scholars. Firstly brief description of the commentaries on *Aṣṭāṅgahṛdaya* by various scholars from different parts of India and then commentaries by Kerala scholars are given below :

1. *Padārthacandrikā* – It is a commentary by Candranandana, son of Ravinandana. He was a native of Kashmir and wrote this at the instance of Sakunadeva, King of Kashmir. He belonged to 10 century AD.[44]

    Padārthacandrikā is by far the earliest available commentary on *Aṣṭāṅgahṛdaya*. It is available in full in manuscript form. Only some portions of it is in print and furnished in the footnote in the extant edition brought out by Harisastry Paradkar. Its Tibetan translation is available in full and is included in the Tanjore collection.[45]

2. *Sarvāṅgasundarī* – It is a commentary available in full and is print by Aruṇadatta, son of Mṛgāṅkadatta.[46] He probably belonged to Bengal and was a great scholar not only in Āyurveda but also in *vyākaraṇa* and other Sanskrit literature. He is identified by some authorities with the lexicographer of the same name. He is assignable to early part of the 12th century AD and he is quoted by Hemādri (13th –14 AD.) His name appears in the commentary of Ḍalhaṇa (11AD) but some scholars doubt its cannotation.[47] Dr. Srikantha Murthy after examining the above points arrived at a conclusion that Aruṇadatta belonged to 10th or 11th AD.[48]

    Sarvāṅgasundarī is a fairly elaborate commentary which explains the meanings with the help of grammar, substantiates with quotations from other texts, and provides synonyms of drugs and even common names for their identification. With these merits it justifies its name and reflects the erudition of its author. There is a popular saying in Malayalam thus:

aṣṭāṅgahṛdayavyākhye

ninnekkāṇātuḷḷannu ñān /

maññaḷeḷlm vayambāyi

karpūram(rāmaccam)? Koṭuveḷiyāy // [49]

Oh, *Aṣṭāṅgahṛdayavyākhya* (*sarvāṅgasundarī*), I am very much worried about your absence. All *maññaḷ* (Turmeric) become *vayampu* (Sweetflag) and all *karpūram* (Camphor) become *koṭuveḷi* (Plumbagoindica).

All synonyms of turmeric denote night and all synonyms of *karpūra* denote moon in *Aṣṭāṅgahṛdaya*. Here *vayampu* has the quality of *tīkṣṇa* (firy) and *koṭuveḷi* is the synonym of *agni* (fire).

This saying brings out *Vipralambhaśṛṅgāra* of a hero as well as the experience of the author in the absence of *sarvāṅgasundarīvyākhyā*. This brings forth the importance of the *Vyākhyā* in understanding *Aṣṭāṅgahṛdaya*.

3. *Āyurvedarasāyana* – It is a work of Hemādri, son of Kāmadeva. He was a Maharastra Brahmin belonging to *vatsagotra*. He was the chief minister and adviser (*dharmādhikārin*) to King Mahādeva (1260 – 71) and his son Ramachadra (1271 –1309), the Yādava rulers of Devagiri.[50]

   Āyurvedarasāyana is not available in full, but available only for *sūtrasthāna, nidānasthāna*, first six chapters of *cikitsāsthāna* and all chapters of *kalpa-siddhisthāna* and these have been printed.

4. *Nidānacintāmaṇi*—It is a commentary on *nidānasthāna* of *Aṣṭāṅgahṛdaya*. It is a work of a scholar by name Toḍaramalla Kanhaprabhu, son of Mahāvaidya Beimadeva Prabhu and Samambika.[51]

   This commentary has been printed in Harisastry Pravadkor's edition. Its date is not yet decided, most likely it belongs to 14 –15 century AD.

5. *Tatvabodha* – This commentary is only for the *uttarasthāna* of *Aṣṭāṅgahṛdaya* by Sivadāsasena, son of Anantasena, who was the court physician to Barbak Shah, Sultan of Bengal (1457-1474). This commentary was probably written in 1500 AD and is available in print.

6. *Vāgbhaṭamaṇḍana* – It is not a commentary but a compendium intended to defend the text from certain objections. A scholar by name

Soura Vidyādhara finds many faults in *Aṣṭāṅgahṛdaya* and abuses its author Vāgbhaṭa. Bhaṭṭanarahari, son of Bhaṭṭa śivadeva refutes all the objections of Vidyādhara and defends Vāgbhaṭa. Both the accuser and the defender support their arguments with quotations from other authoritative texts. Thus *Vāgbhaṭamaṇḍana* is a polemic work of a high standard and only one of its kind in Āyurveda literature. It is tentatively assigned to 15 AD.[52]

Apart from these, the commentaries known have been written Bhaṭṭāra Hariścandra (600 AD), Himadatta (8 AD) Jejjaṭa (9AD) Indu (12-13 AD) and some others have not been traced so far.

Keralite commentaries on *Aṣṭāṅgahṛdaya*

1. *Hṛdayabodhika* – It is a commentary by Śrīdāsapaṇḍita who was a disciple of a scholar by name Vāsudeva. Only the first portion of this commentary (*sūtra, śarīra* and *nidānasthānas*) has been printed. This commentary is brief and furnishes Malyalam equivalents to the name of drugs. Śrīdāsapaṇḍita quotes another commentary by name Vyākhyāsāra written by student of his own teacher, Vāsudeva. Both *Hṛdayabodhika* and *Vyākhyāsāra* have been provided with a short summary in Malayalam called *Alpabuddhiprabodhana* written by a scholar named Śrīkaṇṭha. Śrīdāsapaṇḍita belonged to early part of 14ᵗʰ century and Śrīkaṇṭha to the later part of it. [53]

2. *Pāṭhya*– This commentary is considered to be older one which had been followed by succeeding interpretations. Vaṭakkumkūr in his *Keralīya Samskṛta Sāhitya Caritram* points out that from the definition given by the author itself one can infer the quality of *Pāṭhya*, as follows :

> *upodghātaḥ padam caiva padārthaḥ padavigrahaḥ /*
>
> *cālanā pratyavasthā ca śodhā vyākhyānalakṣaṇam //* [54]

A good commentary needs good introduction, simple words, lucid meanings, simplified words and meanings in compound words, propriety and clarity of expression.

N.V Krishnankutty Varrier in his *Āyurvedacaritram* points out that the author of *vākyapradīpikā* quoted many ślokas from pāṭhya, which shows its authenticity at that time.[55] The author and his date are not known.

3. *Kairalī* - It is a well known commentary considered to be authored by one Pulāmantol Mūsad, one of the Aṣṭavaidias of Kerala. His date and other details are not known. This commentary is only for uttarasthāna of *Aṣṭāṅgahṛdaya* excluding the rasāyana and vājīkaraṇa. Vaṭakkumkūr points out that rasāyana and vājīkaraṇa are not taught to non — brāhmin students and to brāhmin students too after their completion of studies. So this might be reason for the lack of commentaries of the respective chapters.[56] The peculiarity of this interpretation is that it gives the prose order of the ślokas the individual word meanings and Malayalam equivalent names of diseases. So it is very useful to the students of Āyurveda.

4. *Hṛdyā* — This is also a good commentary on *Aṣṭāṅgahṛdaya.* But the date and authorship is not known.

5. *Laḷitā* — This is a commentary on *Aṣṭāṅgahṛdaya* by one Pulāmantol Mūsad. It did not received the recognition it deserved. From the colophon in his work name of his teacher and Guru are available.

> *iti kaṇṭakīphalāndolikālaya*
>
> *vikhyātaśrīnārāyaṇaśarmasūnunā*
>
> *vayaskaraviśiṣṭāgāranamāntaraśobhināghalāvanālaya*
>
> *viśrutanīlakarmaśarmaṇo 'ntevāsināśaṅkaraśarmaṇā*
>
> *viracitāyām lalitākhyāyām aṣṭāṅgahṛdayākhyāyām*.........[57]

The author himself gives the features of this commentary thus:

> *sundaryādiṣvavaiśadyadarthanāmalpacetasām*
>
> *vistārādarthagāmbhīryādvyākhyām kartum yatāmahe /*
>
> *hṛdyendupāṭhyavyākhyānamatabhedapradarśanīm*
>
> *samālambya gabhīrārthām vyākhyām hṛdayabodhikām /*
>
> *nasyādivastiparyantam sūtrasthānām yathāmati*
>
> *vyākhyāsye nīlakaṇṭhasya prasādāt pāṭhyamārgataḥ //* [58]

With blessing of Nīlakaṇṭha, I am going to prepare a commentary on *Aṣṭāṅgahṛdaya* named *Hṛdayabodhika* after examining the predecessors texts like *hṛdya*, *indu* and *pāṭhya* prepared in such a way that will be accessible to an average student.

6. *Vākyapradīpika* – It is written by one Parameśvaran Nambūtiri of Ālattūr village. This information is available from his own statement at the end of *sūtrasthāna* thus:

   itinilātīragatāsvasthagrāmavāsinā   parameśvaradvijottamena   kṛtāyām aṣṭāṅgahṛdayavyākhyāyām   vākyapradīpikāyām   sūtrasthāne   trimśodh yāyaḥ. [59]

   This is the 30th chapter of *sūtrasthāna* in *vākyapradīpikā* of *Aṣṭāṅgahṛdaya* by Ālattūr Parameśvaran Nambūtiri.

7. *Bhāskarīyam* – This commentary is composed by 'Kaṇṇūru Vaidyan Uppoṭṭ Kaṇṇan. Born in Kaṇṇūr in the year 1825 at Kaṇṇūr composed this commentary on 1878.

8. *Sārārthadarpaṇam* – It was composed by Kaikkulaṅṅara Rāma Varrier. He was adept in Āyurveda and Astrology. He was born in 1832 at Kaikkulaṅṅara Varriem and died in 1894.[60]

9. *Aruṇodayam* – It was composed by Kāyikkara P.M Govindan Vaidyan. He has also translated *Aṣṭāṅgahṛdaya* into Malayalam. He was born in 1875 at Chirayankeezhu Taluk and died on 1939. After seeing his mastery over Āyurveda Mahākavi Kumāran Āśān conferred him on the Title *Abhinavavāgbhaṭah.*[61]

10. *Prakāśikā* – It is a commentary on *Aṣṭāṅgahṛdaya* by Dr. Raghvan Thirumulpad. He has commented the *Aṣṭāṅgahṛdaya* in a lucid style even to under stand the beginners of Āyurveda. it deserves special mention because it is accepted as a reference text in Kerala Āyurvedic Colleges. The author has commented on *Aṣṭāṅgasaṅgraha* and *Rasavaiśeṣika* in the same name *Prakāśikā*.

Dr. Raghavan Thirumulppad is well known not only as a physician but also an academician. He was born in Alappuzha district on 20th May 1920 AD as the son of Narayana Iyyer of Chingoli village and Lakshmykkutty Nambisthatiri. After completing Matriculation from Government High School Chalakkudy in 1937, he joined as an employ in Southern Railways. Due to the attack of tuberculosis diseases in 1942 he was compelled to retire from his duties. He returned to Chalakkudy and was attracted to Gandhian principles and joined in that stream. His diseases were cured by Āyurvedic treatment. After that he studied Āyurveda and secured Vaidyabhūṣaṇa certificate after completion of course for 5 years. During his studies he mastered Sanskrit language and Jyotiṣa.

He has composed a large number of works on Āyurveda in Malayalam. *Āyurvedaparicayam*. *Āyurvedadarśanam*, *Aṣṭāṅgadarśanam* are some among them. He wrote commentaries named *Prakāśikā* on *Aṣṭāṅgasaṅgraha*, *Aṣṭāṅgahṛdaya* and *Rasavaiśeṣika* which have been widely used by the students of Kerala Āyurvedic colleges as their reference texts. He occupies the position of a columist *in Ārogyamāsikā,* a publication of *Mathrubhumi* Daily. The awards conferred on him are *Keralapatañjali, Āyurvedaratnam, Paṇḍitaratnam* and *Vaidyabhūṣaṇam.* He got the central Government fellowship for the service rendered by him to the field of Āyurveda.

Apart from these, there are so many commentaries on Āyurveda by scholars like Vayaskara N.S. Musad, and *Āyurvedabhūṣaṇam* M. Keśavan Embrāntiri and V.M. Kuttikrisnamenon etc are available now. From this one can infer that Vāgbhaṭas work has gained great popularity in the succeeding generations.

References

1. K.R Srikantha Murthy, Introduction, *Aṣṭāṅgahṛdaya* (Tr), p.XXII

2. Vāgbhaṭa, *Aṣṭāṅgahṛdaya,* uttarasthāna 40/80

3. *Ibid.,* 40/83

4. Vāgbhaṭa, *Aṣṭāṅgasaṅgraha,* uttarasthāna 50/203-204

5. *Ibid., sūtrasthāna* 1/18

6. K.R Srikantha Murthy, Introduction, *Aṣṭāṅgahṛdaya* (Tr), p. XXII

7. *Ibid.,* XVIII

8. Sachau-*Alberuni's India* Preface; *Ibid.,* XIX

    Aṣṭāṅgahṛdaya - A study

9. *Aṣṭāṅgahṛdaya,* sūtrasthāna 1/1

10. *Ibid.,* 1/3

11. *Carakasamhitā,* sūtrasthāna -1

12. *Aṣṭāṅgahṛdaya,* sūtrasthāna 1/4

13. *Ibid.,* 1/5

14. *Ibid.,* 1/6

15. *Ibid.,* 1/20

16. *Ibid.*

17. Dr. C.K.Ramachandran, *Ārogyamāsikā*, p.8.

18. *Ibid.,* 1/22

19. *Ibid.,* 3/1

20. *Ibid.,* 4/36

21. *Ibid.,* 5/19

22. *Ibid.,* 5/62

23. *Ibid.,* 7/61

24. *Ibid.,* 12/56

25. *Ibid.,* 14/36

26. *Ibid.,* 30/53

27. *Ibid.,* śarīrasthāna 2/8

28. *Ibid.,* 3/2, 3,4

29. *Ibid.,* 6/72

30. *Ibid.,* nidānasthāna 1/1

31. K.R. Srikantha Murthy, *Aṣṭāṅgahṛdaya* (Eng Tr), Vol.II p.3

32. *Supra,* 1/2

33. *Ibid.,* 10/3

34. *Ibid.,* cikitsāsthāna, 22/74

35. *Ibid.,* kalpasiddhisthāna, 6/30

36. *Ibid.,* uttarasthāna, 39/1,2

37. *Ibid.,* 39/181

38. *Ibid.,* 40/79,80

39. *Ibid.,* 40/83, 84

40. *Ibid.,* 40/85

41. *Ibid.,* 40/87

42. *Ibid.,* 40/88

43. *Ibid.,* 40/89

44. Meulenbeld, G.J – *Mādhavanidāna and its chief commentaries* p.402

45. *Ibid.*

46. Aruṇadatta–*sarvāṅgasundaravyākhyā,* Introductory verses, Aṣṭāṅgahṛdaya, sūtrasthāna, 1/1

47. *Ḍalhaṇas Vyākhyā* – sūtrasthāna – kalpasthāna 1/33

48. Srikantha Murthy – Introduction to *Aṣṭāṅgahṛdaya,* p.XXII

49. N.V.K Varrier, 'Keralattinte Āyurvedapāramparyam', *Smaraṇikā* S.S.U.S, Kalady, p.134.

50. Hemādri – Introductory verses of *Āyurveda rasāyana Vyākhyā.*

51. Colophon in the manuscript – Vide introduction to *Aṣṭāṅgahṛdaya,* Harisastry paradkar. Sri Kantha Murthy, Introduction to *Aṣṭāṅgahṛdaya,* p. XXIV

52. Srikantha Murthy, Introduction to *Aṣṭāṅgahṛdaya,* p. XXV

53. Meulenbelb G.J, *Mādhavanidāna* and its chief commentaries, p.430

54. Vaṭakkumkūr – *KSSC,* p.511, Vol.1

55. N.V.K Varrier, *Āyurvedacaritram,* p.345

56. Vaṭakkumkūr, *KSSC,* p.512 Vol.1

57. *Ibid.*

58. *Ibid.,* 513

59. *Ibid.*

60. K.P Sreekumari Amma, *Āyurveda itihāsam* (Ed) Govt. Āyurveda College, Trivandrum.

61. *Ibid.*

Chapter 6

ĀYURVEDIC WORKS BY KERALITE AUTHORS

Apart from the Āyurvedic texts like *Aṣṭāṅgahṛdaya* composed elsewhere, Kerala physicians have followed several works written by Keralite scholars in the practice of Āyurveda. There are twelve independent works on Āyurveda by Keralite authors available now. They are *Bheṣajapaddhati*, *Rasavaiśeṣika*, *Sahasrayoga*, *Tantrasārasaṅgraha*, *Hṛdayapriyā*, *Sukhasādhaka*, *Dhārākalpa*, *Ārogyakalpadruma*, *Aṣṭāṅgaśarīra*, *Bṛhacchārīra*, *Vaidyamanoramā*, and *Kautukacintāmaṇi*. A detailed account of the following is attempted here:

A. *BHEṢAJAPADDHATI*

Bheṣajapaddhati is a short treatise on Āyurveda written by one Puruṣottaman Nambūtiri of Kiḷḷikuruśśimaṅgalam, near Lakkiḍi. The other details of the author are obscure, but it is to be supposed that he was staying with his guru and wrote the book under his directions and guidance.[1] Puruṣottaman Nambūtiri begins the work, paying homage to his Guru and Lord Śiva of the local temple for blessings.

> *śrīmaṅgalaikanilyam bhiṣajāmadhīśam*
>
> *sarvajñamātmagurumapyamṛtāśanānām /*
>
> *śrīnīlakaṇṭhamabhayapradamātmabhāja*
>
> *micchānukūlaphaladam gurumānatosmi //* [2]

> *I salute Śrī Nīlakaṇṭha, my teacher, who is the abode of all auspiciousness, who is the Lord among the physicians, who is omniscient and who is the giver of all fruits as per the aspiration of the disciples like Śiva who is the soul abode of all auspiciousness, who is the best among the physicians who is omniscient, who is the lord of Gods and who fulfills all aspirations of the devotees.*

In the next verse the author pays homage to his *Iṣṭadevatā*, The Lord Viṣṇu, and to his succession of teachers (*ācāryaparamparā*) of Āyurveda along with his immediate teacher

śrīśam padmabhavam prajāpatimaham vāstoṣpatiñcāśvinā-

Vātreyādimunīśvarān kṛtamahātantrāgniveśādikān /

ācāryān praṇipatya vāhaṭamapi śrīnīlakaṇṭham gurum

vakṣye bheṣajapaddhatim guṇanikā siddhyai gurorajñayā // [3]

After having offered my salutations to the Lord of Lakṣmī, Brahman the creator, Indra, Aśvin brothers, the sages Ātreya etc; including Vāhaṭa who have comprised great treatises on Āyurveda and having saluted my Guru Śrī Nīlakaṇṭha, I composed this work called *Bheṣajapaddhati*, on the direction of my teacher in order to attain perfection in the field of Āyurveda.

In the last verse also Puruṣottaman Nambūtiri makes mention of Acyuta, his *iṣṭadevatā,* by whose grace he got the ability to compose this work.

eṣā paddhatiracyutāśrayatayā vāṇī satām sammatā/

doṣaghnī ca bhavennṛṇāmaviduṣām karmaprakāśātmikā // [4]

As this venture is carried out by the grace of Lord Viṣṇu, it will be acceptable to the knowledgeable people. Moreover it will help the ordinary people to get enlightened about the treatment.

Puruṣottaman Nambūtiri being a Sanskrit scholar with poetic talents has no difficulty to give vent to his technical knowledge in beautiful verses. *Bheṣajapaddhati* is a summary of *Aṣṭāṅgahṛdaya* which itself is the most concise Āyurvedic text dealing with all topics. Formerly students had to memorise all the 120 chapters of this *Aṣṭāṅgahṛdaya* but thanks to the efforts of Puruṣottaman Nambūtiri the gist of *Aṣṭāṅgahṛdaya* has been given in *Bheṣajapaddhati*. Noticing this Paṇḍitarājan Tṛkkovil Acyuta Vārrier observe thus:

Perhaps the author predicted the difficulty of the present day students in memorising the whole book and condensed the more important parts in as few verses as possible into four small chapters.[5]

Bheṣajapaddhati contains four small chapters, technically called four *khaṇḍas*. The first *rogavicārakhaṇḍa* (discussion of diseases) consists of sixty-four verses. Among these five verses dealing with the composition of the human body.[6] Then in eight verses the seven *Prakṛtis* (natures)[7] are dealth with. In the next fifteen verses explaining the author explains the symptoms of the *Tridoṣas* (three humours) in both the states of equilibrium and absence of the equilibrium.[8] Then the thirteen verses deals with names and symptoms of diseases.[9] In the next fifteen verses *vikṛtivijñānīya* (knowledge of bad Prognostics)[10] is dealt with.

In short the fundamental principles of Āyurveda mentioned in the *sūtrasthāna*, the *śarīrasthāna* and *nidānasthānas* in *Aṣṭāṅgahṛdaya* are included in this short *khaṇḍa*.

The second *khaṇḍa*, named *Bheṣajavikalpakhaṇḍa* contains thirty-nine verses. Among these the first fifteen verses are devoted to give the properties, *rasa*, (taste) *vīrya*, (efficasy) *vipāka*, (change) and *prabhāva* (potency) of commonly used *dravas* (liquids) and *dravyas* (materials).[11] The next two are devoted to cooked articles of food.[12] *Dravyas* are classified according to their *rasas* (taste) and *guṇas* (qualities) in another eleven verses.[13] The preparation of decoction and other medicines is hinted in three *ślokas*.[14] In the next eight verses *svasthavṛttam*, (routine for health) *ṛtucaryā* (sesonal regments *rogānulpādanīyam* (prevention of diseases) and *mātrātiśīya* (partaking properquantity of food) are concisely dealt with.[15] It can be said that some important portions of *sūtrasthāna* and *kalpasthāna* are thus included in this chapter.

In the third *khaṇḍa* named as *kriyābhedakhaṇḍa* consisting of thirtyone verses the functions of *doṣas, dhātus*, and *malas* are explained briefly. In the examination of the patient importance of *dūtavijñānīyam* (knowledge about the messenger) is stressed.[16] The essence of Āyurveda treatment, *laṅghana, bṛmhaṇa, śodhana and śamana*, the *pañca karmas* and the *upakarmas* are mentioned briefly. Several chapters of *sūtrasthāna* and one in *śarīrasthāna* in the *Aṣṭāṅgahṛdaya* are summarized here.[17]

In the fourth *khaṇḍa* named as *upakramakhaṇḍa* consisting of 101 verses the treatment of *kāyikarogas* is mentioned in the first eightythree verses. Among these sixteen are devoted for fever,[18] four for *raktapitta* (bleeding) and allied diseases,[19] seven for bronchial troubles,[20] eight for *gulma* (abdmonal tumours) [21] and eight for leprosy.[22]

Original verses from *Aṣṭāṅgahṛdaya* are commonly used in the summary. [23] The treatment of certain diseases is given in one or two verses only. Diseases above neck are dealt with in eight verses and other diseases mentioned in Uttarasthāna of *Aṣṭāṅgahṛdaya* in another eight verses.

It can be generally said that the author does not give necessary importance to the treatment of several diseases.

Is *Bheṣajapaddhati* a Kerala work?

There are so many internal evidences to believe that it is a Kerala work authored by a Keralite named Puruṣottaman Nambūtiri. The foremost reason is that Puruṣottaman Nambūtiri has included Vāgbhaṭa also in the guruparamparā and that he used *Aṣṭāṅgahṛdaya* as the basis for his work.[24] Both Vāgbhaṭa and *Aṣṭāṅgahṛdaya* are authentic in Kerala. It can be seen that in some places he adapted verses of *Aṣṭāṅgahṛdaya* according to the environment of Kerala. For example *Aṣṭāṅgahṛdaya* mentions about six *ṛtus*.

> *māsairdvisamkhairmāghādyaiḥ*
>
> *kramāt ṣaḍṛtavaḥ smṛtāḥ /*
>
> *śiśirothavasantaśca*
>
> *grīṣmavarṣaśaraddhimāḥ //*[25]

Beginning with māgha the six combinations of two months, are regarded as six seasons namely *Śiśira, Vasanta, Grīṣma, Varṣa, Śarat* and *Hemanta* respectively.

But three *ṛtus* are mentioned in *Bheṣajapaddhati* in connection with the three doṣas (homours)

> *varṣaśaradvasanteṣu*
>
> *vātapittakaphacchidaḥ /*
>
> *kriyā kāryā viśeṣeṇa*
>
> *vīkṣyā doṣaphalam sadā //*[26]

During the seasons namely, *Varṣa, Śarat* and *Vasanta*, special treatment should be given after examining the *vāta, pitta* and *kapha* of the individual thoroughly.

In the introduction to the text *Bheṣajapaddhati* Paṇḍitarāja Tṛkkovil Acyuta Vārrier says that in the manuscript got from the Tṛkkovil Uzhuttira Vārrier, a few Malayalam verses are seen, which too are included in the text.

niśākatakinellikkāteccipāccotti gopikā

ekanāyakarāmacca mebhiḥ kvātham pramehaham /

nīrūrīvairiteliśūkapuḷikkuruttol

mukhaviḷārpasayumampalari sakāntā /

cemmaṇniśādvayahimadvayamattinīril

saptāhapiṣṭamitu mehagaṇam bhinatti // [27]

The decoction prepared out the following two cure diabetes (1) Turmeric, (2) Water purifying seed, (3) Dry embilic myrobalam (4) Root of the jungle – flame tree (5) Bark of chunga (6) The root of salacia retculatawight (7) The root of aerva lanata, (8) The bark of the root of salacia retculata wight, and (9) Vetiver.

It is remarkable to note that the author quotes the follwing verses from *Sahasrayoga*. [28] *Panaviralkaṭalāṭi cullirambhā*

bhasitasametajalena pālinālum /

azhakilitu nihanti kaññi śopham

harihariyoriva kalmaṣam prasādaḥ // [29]

The solution prepared out of the ashes of the following; flowers of palm, root of the prickly chaff- flower plant, roof of the long leaved berleria, root of the plantain mixed with equal quantities of milk and water cures śopha diseases like the benefits of blessing of god Viṣṇu and Śiva.

This is also a quotation from *Sahasrayoga*. [30]

Mention of coconut oil and the qualities are described in *Bheṣajavikalpakhaṇḍa:*

mūtram rūkṣakaṭuṣṇatīkṣṇalaghu dhānyāmlañca madyāni vā

tailam vātakaphāpaham guru vasā naimbam thatā tauvaram /

airaṇdam kaṭivātajit daśanaśūlaghnaśca kerodbhavam

sarvam vātakaphāpaham śravaṇāsulaghnaśca rājībhavam // [31]

Urine which is *rukṣa* (astringent), *kaṭu* (acrid), *tīkṣṇa* (saltpitre), and laghu (light), rice soup or liquor or gingely oil destroyes all type of diseases, due to *vāta* and *kapha*. *Vasā* (oil taken out of heat) etc. are *guru* (hard) (that is not easily digestable). Neem oil is sour. Castrol oil destroys rheumatic diseases especially of lower region of body. Coconut oil cures tooth ache. Mustard oil destroys all diseases due to *vāta* and *kapha* and cures ear pain.

Also

> *kṣīradrumodarakaravākhadirāsaneṣu*
>
> *jambvarjunadviśabarījatusarjaphenāḥ /*
>
> *kerādripuṣpajavītatagairikādyāḥ*
>
> *patthyādvayendrasuṣavī pramukhāḥ kaṣāyāḥ //* [32]

In the *upakrama khaṇḍa* also there is a reference to coconut as an ingredient of medicine as follows.

> *doṣeṣu sannipatite vivaśe śarīre*
>
> *naṣṭasmṛtau nakhamukhādiṣu taila lepaḥ /*
>
> *sastaśca pānamapi bhodhanamindriyāṇām*
>
> *nasyam supakvamiha kerajanimbajaśca. //* [33]

When the *doṣas* are manifest, the body is in an unconscious state and the memory has failed, the application of gingely oil on the nails, face etc; or the drinking or inhailing of the boiled coconut oil and neem oil are able to bring back the senses to consciousness.

Puruṣottaman Nambūtiri has given a special preparation of medicine with coconut flowers for *asṛgdaram*. He mentions that it is the special medicine of his *guru.*

> *asṛgdare 'pyevamihātimātra*
>
> *pravṛttaraktapraśamāya peyam /*
>
> *japāpayaḥ kerajapuṣpasāram*
>
> *sitāmadhubhyāmiti me gurūktiḥ //* [34]

According to my teacher the excess bleeding due to *asṛgdara* (enlargement of rectum) can be cured by the intake of the decoction prepared out of the flower stalk of red coconut tree, the buds of white Hibiscus added with sugar and honey.

Mention of coconut water for treatment is given in *upakramakhaṇḍa.*

> *kṛcchreṣu pittapavanātmasumūtravṛddhyai*
>
> *kvātham pibellaghu tṛṇātmakapañcamūlaiḥ /*
>
> *sakṣīramājyamapi tairmadhurañca peyam*
>
> *kerāmbunājyatilakairabhiṣecayettam //* [35]

The difficulty in passing urine due to the excess of *vāta* and *pitta* can be cured and the urine can be increased by the consumption of decoction of the following ingredients namely, root of Desmodium, root of psuedathia viscido, poison berry, land caltrops etc. The *dhārā* therapy by using coconut water, ghee or gigely oil is good for this disease.

Again

vātaśleṣmasu dāśamūla salilam

peyamañca dhānyāmlataḥ /

svedaḥ kerajanimbatailavasayā-

bhyaṅgo vyavāyādayaḥ // [36]

The urinary disease arising of the excess of *vāta* and *kapha* element can be cured by the intake of *dasamūlasalīla* or prespiration by rice soup and apply coconut oil or Neem oil or *Vasā* for massage.

Another point suggesting the Keralite authorship is that the manuscript for *Bheṣajapaddhati* has been recovered from Kerala and three verses are given in Malayalam language and another one in *Maṇipravāḷa*. [37]

In the concluding portion of the *Bheṣajapaddhati* it is said that there are some medicines which are not mentioned in basic authentic texts. It seems that those were the special preparation of his Guru. In one of the verses he mentions about *kāyaseka* which is known as *pizhiccil, a* peculiar technique evolved in Kerala Āyurveda.

chinne bhinne ca bhagne vapuṣi nijanijasthānamāyojyasamyag-

bhadhvā sekādi kuryādyadi tu nipatite śeṣagātrāṇi rakṣet. // [38]

When the limps of the body are fractured or broken then the parts are to joined their respective places and bound carefully and *pizhiccil* therapy can be done. If a part of the body is fallen (cut off) then the rest of the limbs should be protected.

Puruṣottaman Nambūtiri used the word *aśana* for eating. This is a word commonly used in Kerala for *āhāra* (food), while describing *Dinacaryā* (daily routine). It is interesting here to note that Kerala 'cākyārs' used this word abundantly and there is a particular topic named *aśana* in *Kūṭiyāṭṭam.*

uthāyoṣasi śuddha ātmavihitam smṛtvātha kṛtvā harim /

natvā snānamathāsanañca śayanādīni svakāle bhajet // [39]

After waking up very early in the morning, do the following regularly in each day. (1) Pray to Hari, (2) think about one's own duties, (3) then take bath and food and go to bed at the proper time.

A few ślokas from this text and a few from the standard recipes prevalent in Kerala are reproduced as such.

In the last but one verse Puruṣottaman Nambūtiri says that the work is based upon *Aṣṭāṅgahṛdaya*.

> *bheṣajāni suvijñeyānyaṣṭāṅgahṛdaye nṛṇām*
>
> *mano 'nayā viśatyasminnityeṣā paddhatismṛtā //* [40]

Primarily one should have thorough understanding of medicines prescribed in *Aṣṭāṅgahṛdaya;* and later one can enter into this text *'Bheṣajapaddhati'*

Dr. C.R Agnives after examining the medicines prescribed in this text observes that the tablets like *nīrūryādiguḷikā* mentioned in this are prevalent only in Kerala. This also conforms to the view that it is a Keralite work. Most of the medicines prescribed in this text have been using by the Āyurvedic physicians of Kerala for common diseases like Diabetics, and fever. etc.,

From the above evidences it can be categorically concluded that Puruṣottaman Nambūtiri is a Keralite. He is not only a physician but also a master of Sanskrit language. He has abridged many *Aṣṭāṅgahṛdaya* ślokas in lucid and simple Sanskrit language with out loosing the essence.

B. *RASAVAIŚEṢIKA*

Rasavaiśeṣika is a short treatise on Āyurveda written by one *Bhadantanāgārjuna* of first century AD.[41] N.V Krishnankutty Varrier in his *Āyurvedacaritram* points out that he got an opportunity to go through the edition of the text from Trivandrum Sanskrit series and the editor of the text Kolatheri Sankara Menon mentioned that the date of the author as 5th A.D and the date of the interpreter *Nṛsimha* as 8th AD.[42] Nothing definite can be said on this matter.

The text available now was published in July 1993 with the *Prakāśikā* commentary by Dr. Raghavan Tirumulppad through Vaidyaratnam Āyurveda College Taikkattussery, Ollur. Actually it seems to have be composed for giving theoretical foundation to *Rasaśāstra* in Āyurveda. It is interesting here to note that the author does not use the term *Rasavaiśeṣika* anywhere in the text. But from Nṛsimha's commentary on *Rasavaiśeṣika*, one can infer that the name of the text is *Rasavaiśeṣika*.[43]

Is Bhadanta Nāgārjuna a Buddhist monk?

The text Rasavaiśeṣika begins with the aphorism atha ataḥ ārogyaśāstram vyākhyāsyāmaḥ (Then I am going to deal with Āyurveda)

Here it is remarkable to note that Bhadanta Nāgārjuna does not use benedictory verse of traditional nature (*maṅgalaśloka*) in the beginning. This may lead to a conclusion that he is a Buddhist. Dr. Raghavan Thirumulppad while commenting on the text suggested that Bhadanta Nāgārjuna belongs to Buddhist clan.[44] He derived the term *Bhadanta* thus: The term *Bhadanta* is derived from the root *Bhad* which means auspicious. Hence it denotes a Buddhist monk. Moreover the derivation, *bhāni iva prakāśamānāḥ dantāḥ yasya saḥ* (one who posseses teeth that shine like stars) also lead to the same conclusion because Bhadanta Nāgārjuna may be a Buddhist monk who abstained from the sensual pleasures like *tāmbūlacarvaṇa*. Moreover Nāgārjuna is a name popularly used by Buddhists. Hence it is safer to conclude that Bhadanta Nāgārjuna was a Buddhist.

The *Bhāṣyakāra* Nṛsimha is also a Buddhist because while commenting on the opening verse Nṛsimha does not give the meaning 'auspicious'to the word *atha*. There is a common practice among the commentators to interpret *athaśabda* in the sense of auspeciousness:

> *oṅkāraścāthaśabdaśca*
>
> *dvāvetau brahmaṇaḥ purā /*
>
> *kaṇtham bhitvā viniryātau*
>
> *tena māṅgalikāvubhau //*

Oṅkāra and *atha* words are auspicious because they emerged out of the throat of Brahman.

Further Nṛsimha ends his *Bhāṣya* with a statement :

> *Nirvāṇam paramam sukham*

The greatest of all pleasures is the stage of *nirvāṇa* or liberation. This also conforms to the view that Nṛsimha was a Buddhist.[45]

130

RASAVAIŚEṢIKA – AN ANALYSIS

The text consists of 485 Aphorisms divided in to four chapters. It contains detailed discussion of *dravya, rasa, guṇa, vīrya, vipāka* and *karma*.[46] The above six are accepted as six *padārthas.* (categories) of Āyurveda.

The first chapter consists of 171 aphorisms. The first four aphorisms put forward the nature of the subject presented in the text. Then in the next three aphorisms Nāgārjuna explains how these six *padārthas* become the cause for health and diseases. After that the nature and characteristics of six *padārthas* are described. It is interesting to note that there is a reference to *viṣakanya* in the 21st *sūtra.* In olden days *viṣakanyas* were widely used by the kings to kill enemies.

Dr. Raghavan Thirumulpad while describing the qualities of medicine interprets the aphorism *daivapratīghātāt* [47] thus: Here *daiva* means demons because the medicines cure the disease caused by the demons. He quotes a śloka to substantiate this:

> *varjayanti yathāraṇyam sasimham mṛgapakṣiṇah/*
>
> *varjayanti grahāstadvat sauṣadham sūtikāgṛham //* [48]

The Demons abandon that house which is provided with medicine like the lower animals abandoning the forest in which the lion resides.

But this interpretation seems to be not so correct. So far as the semantic aspect is concerned, nowhere in Sanskrit language *daiva* is used in the sense of demon. Moreover it is against the spirit of Veda where gods are also described as inflicting diseases on men. And there was a time in ancient days when people believed that disease were the result of wrong deeds done by them. So it is better to interpret the daiva as fate.

The second chapter consists of 123 aphorisms. The first 22 aphorisms establish the separate existence of *dravya* from other five *padārthas*. In the following aphorisms five basic elements of living beings and the medicinal material on earth are dealt with in detail.

The third chapter consists of 116 aphorisms. The first 72 aphorisms discuss the nature of *rasa* in detail. Then in the following aphorisms the *mātra* (quantity) recommended for various stages of diseases is prescribed. In the 61st aphorism

Bhandanta Nāgārjuna categorically states that among other *pramāṇas, āgama* is the most important.

> *Tasmāt viśeṣeṇa āgama eva*
>
> *Pramāṇam cikitsāyām. //* [49]

āgama pramāṇa is very important among *pramāṇas* so far as treatment is concerned.

There is a similar attitude accepted by Vāgbhaṭa in the *vājīkaraṇa* chapter of *Aṣṭāṅgahṛdaya* :

> *idamāgamasiddhatvāt*
>
> *pratyakṣaphaladarśanāt /*
>
> *mantravat samprayoktavyam*
>
> *na mīmāṃsyam kathañcana. //* [50]

Since these information described in this text are approved by the ancient scriptures and since the benefits (accuring by following them) are perceptible (noticeable clearly with in a short time) these are to be administered like sacred hymns without any discussion (of their efficacy)

The fourth chapter consists of 73 aphorisms. This chapter generally deals with *svasthavṛtta, āturavṛtta,* etc. in detail. The *pramāṇas* accepted in Āyurveda are given as follows:

> *pratyakṣānumānopamānāgamarthāpatti sambhavāḥ pramāṇāni /* [51]

pratyakṣa (perception) anumāna (inference) upamāna (similarity) āgama (the tradition of forefathers regarding medicine.) arthāpatti (assumption) and sambhava (probability) are the six pramāṇas.

Generally Āyurveda accepts three *pramāṇas* perception, inference and *āptavākya.* The *upamāna, arthāpatti* and *sambhava* are included in the above three.

In the following verse *padacatuṣṭaya* (the four elements necessary for the successful treatment) is mentioned.

> *Dravyāturopasthāyakabhiṣajām sampadamapekṣate*
>
> *siddhiḥkarmaṇaḥ. /* [52]

medicine, patient, nurse and doctor are the four requisite elements for successful treatment.

The text concludes with the aphorism :

Karmaṇaśca siddhau sarvārthasiddhiḥ /

The effective treatment leads one to attain all objectives in life.

Is *Rasavaiśeṣika* a Kerala work?

N.V. Krishnankutti Varrier mentiones *Rasavaiśeṣika* as a Kerala work in his *Āyurvedacaritram.*[53] Dr. Raghavan Thirumulppad is also of the same view. He puts forward the following arguments to prove this 1) The original text of *Rasavaiśeṣika* is discovered from Ciraṭṭamaṇṇu Illam near Kottayam District. Ullūr has mentioned this illam as one of the branches of *aṣṭavaidya* clan. The text was first published by Kolatteri Sankara Menon on April 1928. It was later on republished with elaborate commentaries by Muthusvami on October 1976. 2) The text was not popular among other physicians outside Kerala. Moreover an aphorism from *Rasavaiśeṣika* is quoted in *Hṛdayabodhika*, a Keralite commentary on *Aṣṭāṅgahṛdaya.*[54] Dr. Raghavan Thirumulppad shows the quotation in Ḍalhaṇas commentary from *Rasavaiśeṣika*: *saptadoṣataḥ saptaguṇataḥ iti nāgārjunācāryoktatvāt.*[55] However except this one all other materials available are in favour of believing that it is a Kerala work.

C. SAHASRAYOGA OR CIKITSĀSĀRASARVASVA

It is a collection of around 1000 *yogas* (Combinations or recipes) of medicines including the special preparations of Kerala. Eventhough it is a Sanskrit work it also contains certain stray verses in Malayalam. The *Sahasrayoga* text available now is edited by Ara vattazhikattu. K.V. Krisnan Vaidyar and Anekkalilil. S. Gopalapillai published it through Vidyarambham publications Alappuzha. The present text also carries a commentary named *Sujanapriya* by the authors in Malayalam language. In the preface to the text the editors declare that the text is edited with an aim to enrich the knowledge of Āyurvedic physicians and give an understanding to the common mass about the medicinal materials around them.[56] The author of the work is not known. It can be assumed that the date of the composition of the work may not be prior to 15th century A. D. on the ground that the text contains the treatment of Syphilis which is a disease carried here by the Portuguese travellers. The medicine prescribed for Syphilis is given as follows:

cukkum tippaliyoṭu nallamulakum mukkā kariñjīrakam

colkkoṇṭoru varaṭṭumaññaḷuluvānalpavumenniṅṅane /

okkekkoṇṭu kaṣāyamākki niyatam sevikkilenne keṭum

muṣkum kāṭṭi ñeḷiññuvarunnoru parangikkammenen tozhare // [57]

The Syphilis can be cured by the regular use of decoction with honey prepared out of the following ingredients. Dry ginger, Indian long pepper, chilly and, Triphala fruits (Chebutic, Embilic and Belliric).

The text begins with the recipe (*yoga*) of the medicine used in the treatment of common fever thus :

ghanacandanaśuṇṭhyambu

parpaṭo śīrasādhitam /

śītam tebhyo hitam toyam

pācanam tṛṭjvarāpahaḥ // [58]

The water boiled with nut grass root, sandal, dry ginger, hedyotis, plectranthus, and vetiver cures fever if it is taken after cooling. It increases digestion and appetite.

It is remarkable to note that this medicine is commonly used among Keralites as *gṛhavaidya* (home medicine) in the name of *ṣaḍaṅgam kaṣāya*. This text contains a large number of medicines prepared out of medicinal materials easily available in Kerala. An example is cited here to substantiate it from the context of treatment of bleeding thus:

nāḷikeraprasūnairvā

japayā balayāpi vā /

jambūvalkalena vā siddhaḥ

kvāthasṛgdaranāśakaḥ // [59]

The decoction prepared out of any one of the following cures *asṛgdara* (bleeding) the coconut flower, the *sida* and the bark of Jamun tree.

It can be seen that there are a lot of medicines prepared out of the product of coconut tree. This also attests the Kerala origin of the text. Some of the examples are cited below for illustration.

nāḷikerasya puṣpāṇām

nūtanānām rasam pibet // [60]

The intake of the decoction prepared out of the stalk of fresh coconut flower cures bleeding. And

gopīcūrṇam pibet prātaḥ

nāḷikera jalena vā /

pradaram praharatyāśu

viṣeṣātraktapittajit // [61]

The drinking of tender coconut water mixed with dried powder of the roots of country *sarasaparilla* for one day in the morning cures *pradara* (a kind of bleeding).

It also contains the preparation of *vāyuguḷikā*[62] a remedial tablet for gas troubles, *puḷiṅkuzhampu*[63] etc; which are some special preparations of Kerala not seen in the *samhitā* texts of Āyurveda.

The text also contains the preparation of *ariṣṭa, āsava, ghṛta*, and the special medicines for the treatment of poison in detail. It is interesting here to note that this text gives thirteen *hastivargas* (*ottamūḷi*) remedial measures to cure ailments caused by over consumption of food as follows:[64]

CAUSE OF INDIGESTION	REMEDY
1. Black gram	Gingly oil
2. Vegetable leaves	Lemon juice
3. Jack fruit	Ginger (dried)
4. Ghee	Salt water
5. Peas	Chilly powder in butter milk
6. Milk	Indian long pepper (*tippali*)
7. Mango	Coconut milk / Salt water
8. Banana	Crystal salt
9. Dried or half cooked food	Sindhu salt *(induppu)*
10. Jaggery	Rice powder in ghee
11. Horse gram	Butter cream
12. Decayed rice	Hogweed (*tazhutāma*)
13. Chilly	Milk

Several types of purification processes for various metals used for medical purposes are also given in the text. The purification process of a metal namely, iron is quoted below for illustration:

> *urukkulayiliṭṭādyam pazhuppiccatu morilum*
>
> *nalleṇṇayilumennalla gomūtrattilumādarāt /*
>
> *arikkāṭiyilum mukki rākippinnepoticcuṭan*
>
> *ñāvalttolirasam tanniluraccchiṭṭatuṇakkaṇam //* [65]

For the purification of iron, it should be put in the furnace and heated to red colour and soaked into the following viz. butter milk, gingerly oil, urine of a cow, rice soup one after another. Then it should be rubbed to become powder and then grinded and dried in the juice of the bark of jammun tree.

The text ends with *guṇapāṭha* (qualities) of dravyas in general in Malayalam language.

D. *TANTRASĀRASAṄGRAHA*

Tantrasārasaṅgraha or *Viṣanārāyaṇīyam* was written by one scholar Nārāyaṇa who is considered to be one of the top-ranking men well versed in these type of subjects like toxicology in Kerala. He is believed to have lived in 15th or 16th century A.D.[66] Other details about his life and works are not known.

Tantrasārasaṅgraha is a Tāntrik work. The text available now is edited by Dr. Duraisvami Ayyengar through Chaukhamba Sanskrit Pratisthan, New Delhi.The author points out that *tāntric* remedial principles and medicines are not contrary to each other but according to *arsic* viewpoints they are concomitant.

> *sṛṣṭiśca pralayaścaiva daivatānām tathārcanam*
>
> *sādhanam caiva sarveṣām puraścaraṇamevaca /*
>
> *ṣaḍkarmasādhanam caiva dhyānayogaścaturvidhaḥ*
>
> *saptabhirlakṣaṇairyuktam āgamam tāntrikam viduḥ. //* [67]

A *tantra* consists of seven subjects – the creation, the annihilation, the worship of the Gods, the attainment of all objects, repetition of the mantra, attaining perfection in six practices and the four fold meditation.

The author Nārāyaṇa describes all these subjects except the first.

The title *Tantrasārasaṅgraha*

Tantrasārasaṅgraha is the Tittle of the work which is published from Chaukhambha Sanskrit Pratisthan, Delhi. But according to a vague popular version its name is said to be *Viṣanārāyaṇīya*. There is a very popular and widely read classical work in Kerala called *Nārāyaṇīya,* written by Melputtūr Nārāyaṇabhaṭṭatiri. Almost all manuscripts of this Tantrik work, contains the name *Nārāyaṇīya* written in the beginning, at the end of each paṭala and also in the colophon. The people who took *viṣacikitsā* as their profession and who were specially interested in studying this book were reading only up to such chapters ie from one to ten, which deal with Toxicology exclusively and did not take interest in the other greater part of the work containing other subjects. The professional people added the word *Viṣa* before the *Nārāyaṇīya* to distinguish it from the *Nārāyaṇīya* of Melputtūr Nārāyaṇa Bhaṭṭa.

Dr. Duraiswami Ayyengar in his preface to the work points out thus: "This is a (*Viṣanārāyaṇīya*) misconstrued and misapplied name." He put forward the following arguements. First of all the author does not give any hint in the book as *Viṣanārāyaṇīya*. Secondly the chapter from one to ten only deal with the subject is toxicology (*viṣavaidya*). These ten paṭalas form less than one third of the whole work. There is one Manuscript in Malayalam script which contains only up to 10th paṭala. This shows that *viṣacikitsakas* of Kerala do not care to read or write beyond the portion they wanted, of this book. Thirdly the subject *agadatantra* is found to be incomplete even in the portion (in ten chapters) set a part for it as there is no description of herbal and mineral poisons (*sthaviraviṣa*) any where in the book. Dr. Duraiswami Ayyengar observes;

So none, with critical eyes, will agree to call this as a book on *agadatantra* (Toxicology) observed with our open eyes, except No. 3837, bears the name *Viṣanārāyaṇīya*. We are surprised to note that some one (with what motive we do not know) has prefixed two letters *vi* and *ṣa* to the name *Nārāyaṇīya* and *Vaidyam* in the opening page and also clearly post-fixed the word *Viṣavaidya* at the end of the work also just above the line of Colophon after *iti nārāyaṇīya* in the Library copy No. R3837 and this addition of words in two places seems to be entirely spurious [68]

Then Dr. Duraiswami Ayyengar points out various reasons to attest the name *Tantrasārasaṅgraha* accepted by himself.The author himself states in his introductory verses that he has collected all the important materials (*Sārasaṅgraha*) from several *tāntrik* works such as *Śikhā-Yoga-Gārgya, Mahākāla,* etc. and complied this work.

> *Yāvatsāmarthyamāsmabhiḥ sarvalokahitaiṣibhiḥ*
>
> *Sikhāyogaditantrebhyaḥ kriyate sārasaṅgrahaḥ //* [69]

A brief digest is prepared by taking the material from *śikhā, yoga,* etc by me to the best of my ability with the intension of doing good to all people.

Further the author proposes another name also giving due importance to the subject that he deals with in the whole work. There are six different *tāntrika* subjects described in different chapters of this book. The first ten paṭalas are devoted for the subject *viṣa.* In the next four *paṭalas* the author has given an account of the subject *grahapīḍas* and their treatments. The mental disease *unmāda* is also included in this portion. Then two *paṭalas* (15th and 16th) describe various painful bodily ailments and *tāntrika* treatment for them and this subject is specified there as *āmayadhvamsa.* The next curious subject is a mischievous spiritual (magic) like deed of certain persons, say evil minded, which is called, *kṛtya* in Sanskrit; such evil deeds come under the term *kṣudra*; these *kṣudras* and their remedies can be read in the 17th and 18th *paṭalas* under the tittle of *kṣudradhvamsa.* The 19th *paṭala* explains to satisfy some people having interest in materialism and inquisitiveness in conjuring art etc. this subject is called *narma* or *vinoda.* The whole part ie of thrteen *paṭalas,* is entirely devoted for *kāmikakarmas.* In this portion the author comprehensively expresses the *mantras* and the devotional aspirations towards all the dieties with their ultimate effects.

Dr. Duraiswami Ayyengar suggests that the *kāmikakarma* portion is really larger than the *viṣa* portion. So one can reasonably name this book as *kāmika tantra.* The author calls it as *kāmika tantra* in 3rd verse.

> *viṣagrahāmayadhvamsāḥ kṣudram marma ca kāmikam*
>
> *iti ṣaṭkārmikam tantrametat siddhidvayāspadam //* [70]

The text deals with all the affairs of human body and mind originated either by material or spiritual causes. The author expresses this idea in one of his concluding passages that it can be named as *Nārāyaṇīyasarvamantrārthakośa.* Thus the author has used three names-1) *Tantrasārasaṅgraha* 2) *Ṣaṭkārmikatantra* and 3) *Sarvamantrārthakośa*. Among the three names the first is the most comprehensive compendious and compatible and it is the name that the author mentions first in the beginning of the work and it is proper to choose *Tantrasārasaṅgraha* as the name of the work.It seems to be more logical to accept this name *Tantrasārasaṅgraha* because it treats various topics under one head.

Tantrasārasaṅgraha is also edited by Dr. N.V.P.Unithiri with one *Mantravimarśinī* commentary by Svarṇagrāma Vāsudeva and published from Calicut Univeresity. The details of the commentary is given as follows in the following.

Mantravimarśinī – A commentary on *Tantrasārasaṅgraha*

It is a commentary on *Tantrasārasaṅgraha* by Svarṇagrāma Vāsudeva. The text *Tantrasārasaṅgraha* with the commentary is edited by Dr.N.V.P Unithiti from Calicut University in Nov. 2002 in two series No.15 and 16. Dr. N.V.P Unithiri points out that the verse forming the Colophon to each chapter clearly shows that the title of the commentary is *Mantravimarśinī* and the author is Vāsudeva. The verse from the end of the last chapter is quoted to prove this

> *evam mantravimarśinyām*
>
> *śrīmannārāyaṇīyake /*
>
> *vāsudevaparāmṛṣṭam*
>
> *dvātrimśatpaṭalam gatam //* [71]

Thus in *Mantravimarśinī* of Vāsudeva on *Śrīmannārāyaṇīya* the thirty second *paṭala* comes to an end.

Mantravimarśinī commentary explains all the difficult passages in the text. It gives almost all the mantras in *Tantrasārasaṅgraha* in metrical form, probably for the purpose of easy recollection. The author substantiates his views from various authentic works. Dr.N.V.P Unithiri after examining it from the linguistic point of view proves that it a Keralite work.[72]

It is remarkable to note that at the end of the text edited by Dr. N.V.P Unithiri, there are five indices which give the botanical names of medicines, Malayalam and Tamil equivalents of Sanskrit terms and the *Ślokānukramaṇī* which are very useful to the students of Āyurveda.

E. *HṚDAYAPRIYA*

This work is composed by Pāccumūttatu of Vaikkam. The contribution of Vaikkam Pāccumūttatu deserves special mention in the field of Āyurveda. Vaikkam Pāccumūttatu not only composed two important works on Āyurveda namely *Hṛdayapriya* and *Sukhasādhaka* but also composed many works in Sanskrit and Malayalam. His disciple Kaviyūr Parameśvaran Mūttatu instituted Trivandrum Āyurveda College in the year 1886 under his direction.

Author — His Date and Personal Details

Vaikkam Pāccumūttatu or Parameśvara was a native of Vaikkam. He belonged to Śivadvija community of Kerala. He held the office of Vaṭṭappaḷḷi Sthānika attached to the Śiva temple at Sucīndram. Dr. K.K Raja suggests (1816-1883) as the date of Vaikkam Pāccumūttatu' and also that he becomes the *sthānin* of Vaṭṭappaḷḷi in the year 1870AD.[73] Vaikkam Pāccumūttatu lived for 69 years from the Malayalam era 989-1058 (1814-1883).[74] But Subrahmaṇyam Mūttatu the disciple of Vaikkam Pāccumūttatu in the biography at the beginning to the text *Sukhasādhaka* mentions Vaikkam Pāccumūttatu's date as 1806 AD.[75] Vaṭakkumkūr Rāja Rāja, Ullūr S. Parameśvara Iyyer are of the view of the former. Dr. Raghavan Thirumulppad after examining the (kali chronogram) of the birth and death of the Vaikkam Pāccumūttatu *jñāniguṇalabdhisoyam* and *pūjyastrinetradṛṣṭam* opines that these dates were 1814 -1883 AD[76] So this view can be accepted as authentic. Further Sāmba Śiva Śāstri in the preface to the text declares that -

My friend Vāsudevaśarma points out the date of Vaikkam Pāccumūttatu as 1814 —1883, who is descendant of from the author . . . . supply me with a copy of the autobiography of the author written by his own hand and hence the statements found there in may be taken to be perfectly reliable.[77]

His Life

Vaikkam Pāccumūttatu was born in a Brahmin family at Vaikkam. He then followed his family profession of worshipping in a temple for six years along with his uncle Kuññuṇṇi in the village of Tiruppurayattu. During this period he learnt preliminary Sanskrit text *Śrīrāmodanta* from his uncle. At the age of seventeen he lost his uncle, his only guardian and teacher, which event deprived him of learning more of Sanskrit. Meanwhile he learnt painting from Nallūrkkandi Nambūtiri, a priest in the temple at Vaikkam. Then he studied *paṭhaka* from Veccūru Tevalakkāṭṭ Mūttatu and performed it in festivals in various temples and earned some money. At the age of twenty-three he resumed his Sanskrit studies. He learnt Vyākaraṇa texts *Siddhāntakaumudī* and *Tattvabodhinī* from Koṭuṅṅallūr Vidvān Tampurān. He became an adept in various disciplines like *sāhitya, nyāya, vyākaraṇa* and *jyotiṣa* within a short period. He led an austere life observing all the religious rites with scrupulous reverence and acquired a remarkably high order of proficiency in Vyākaraṇa. At the age of thirty he was caught with a terrible skin disease. In order to recover himself from this malady, he went through a course of ascetic discipline worshipping his guardian deity at Vaikkam. There was no sign of abatement of the disease for a long time. He consulted a number of doctors with the object of learning the course of his illness, but was not satisfied with their answers. He now made up his mind to make a study of the science of Āyurveda himself and with the help of his father obtained thorough mastery of that science soon. He then happened to meet the Vaṭaśśeri Nambūtiri, a great *Māntric* teacher and learned from him a long course of prayer and worship.

In 1020 Malayalam Era he was attacked by small pox. During his penance he obtained a direct vision of the deity and in course of time got himself cured of the disease. His fame as a great scholar and physician now spread throughout the land and requisition for his services from people came heavily on him so much so he was not allowed to remain in one place for a single day. Vaikkam Pāccumūttatu tripped all through Travancore, Cochin and neighboring places leading a life of service meeting with due appreciation from all over the country. He was recipient of special honors from three successive Mahārājas of Travancore namely Utrāṭam Tirunāḷ, Āyilyam Tirunāḷ, and Vaiśākham Tirunāḷ.

With the object of perpetuating the fruits of his long study and laborious researches Vaikkam Pāccumūttatu wrote a number of valuable works as desired by people who liked shorter treatises in preference to extensive ancient works. This is as given in at the end of *Hṛdayapriya.*

> *kṛcchrānuṣṭhānabhārairagadasamudayairdurlabhairmiśracihnaiḥ*
>
> *vistīrṇāt pustakaughāt pracakitamanasāmprārthanāt sampraṇītaḥ /*

'grantho'sau lokahṛdyaḥ' kalitabahurujālakṣaṇaḥ siddhayogo

bhūyādayuḥsukhānāmayasucaritadaḥ śambhuvat svāśritānām // [78]

Let this book called *Hṛdayapriya* bring longevity, pleasure, health and good conduct to those who consult it just as Śambu who grants longevity, pleasure, and health, as it gives the diagnosis of various diseases. This short book is written on the request of those who are frightened by the multitude of elaborate (large) books which prescribed (stipulate) very highly different practices of group of medicines which are scarce and confused.

The chronogram *grantho'sau lokahṛdyah* in the above verse shows the Kalidina on which the work is said to have been completed which is 29th Dhanu 1040 of the M.E and it is clear therefore that the author wrote his present work with his mature intellect; when he was past fifty. This work became popular even during the lifetime of the author and has since been used to daily study by all Āyurvedic students and teachers of Kerala.

Hṛdayapriya - Contents

Hṛdayapriya is a short treatise on Āyurveda rendered in simple Sanskrit *kārikas* (verses). The method of lucid presentation and preciseness of the author can be infered from this text. The author himself states that he had used many *Aṣṭāṅgahṛdaya* ślokas in his work and simplified them for the understanding of the average students:

prāyenāṣṭāṅgahṛdayaproktaiḥ padyairnavairapi /

tadarthānusṛtaiḥ kurve bālānām hṛdayapriyam // [79]

The text begins with a verse (śloka) paying homage to Śiva the presiding deity of Vaikkam temple.

śrīmadvyāghrālayādhīśam bhiṣaktamamupāsmahe

rogān jvarādīn rāgādīn jitvā diśati yassukham // [80]

I offer my prayer to the deity at Vaikkam temple and Lord of physicians who destroys the diseases such as fever and gives happiness by helping to conquer passion etc.

From the *kārikā* (verse) at the end of the first *khaṇḍa* of *Hṛdayapriyaḥ* one can infer that the name of the text is *Hṛdayapriyaḥ* and the author is Parameśvara. Thus:

nityam śrīparameśvarasya bhajatā vyāghrālayādhīśituḥ

pādābjam parameśvareṇa śivabhūdevanvayodbhūtinā /

samkṣipte hṛdayapriye prakalitaḥ khaṇḍotra kalpābhidho

modāyāstu guṇetaro vimṛśatām mātsaryavarjam satām // [81]

The first section called *Kalpakhaṇḍa* comes to an end in the work called *Hṛdayapriya* which is a brief account of Āyurveda composed by Parameśvara who is born in the family of *śivadvijas* of (Vaikkam) and who ever cherishes and praises the feet lotus of Śrī Parameśvara the lord of the Śiva temple at Vaikkam. This is for the delight of the learned who make an assessment of the work without any influence of jealousy.

Hṛdayapriya consists of four chapters which are technically called *khaṇḍas*. Of the four *khaṇḍas* in the work, the first three deal with the substance of *Aṣṭāṅgahṛdaya* while the last deals with the essential medicinal *yogas* recognised by other *ācāryas* especially in Kerala. Sāmbaśivaśāstrī in the preface to the work *Hṛdayapriya* observes thus:

Vāhaṭācārya finding the gradual diminuation in the tenure of human life, the inability of people to study the extensive medical treatise of ancient authors and the consequent disappearance of the vast Āyurvedic lore, wrote a short treatise named *Aṣṭāṅgahṛdaya*; similarly Parameśvara who came centuries after Vāhaṭācārya, fearing that the succeeding generation would be in still worse condition wrote for their benefit a simpler treatise on medicine named *Hṛdayapriya*.[82]

Parameśvara condenses the *Aṣṭāṅgahṛdaya* which dealt with six sthānas viz, *sūtra, śarīra, nidāna, cikitsā, kalpa*, and *uttara*, and which on the whole contain 120 chapters, into three *khaṇḍas* consisting of forty eight chapters. Further the author added a *khaṇḍa* named *yogakhaṇḍa* containing twelve chapters dealing with the medical *Yogas* (recipes) prevailing among Kerala physicians. Thus Vaikkam Pāccumūttatu like a modern Vāhaṭācārya has given us a complete treatment of medicine in 60 (48+12) chapters with the *yoga* as an additional subject. The author has a thorough grasp of the subject and complete mastery over the language. He shows his high regard for Vāgbhaṭa by adopting in his work and mostly dealing with the subject matter on the lines of the latter, as stated explicitly in

Prāyenāṣṭāṅgahṛdayaproktaiḥ / [83]

Most of them (subject) according to *Aṣṭāṅgahṛdaya*.

This is the path followed by learned men in olden days which can be inferred from *Abhinavabhāratī* of *Abhinavagupta.*

ūrdhvordhvamāruhya yadarthatatvam

dhī paśyati śrāntimavedayanti /

phalam tadādyaiḥ parikalpitānām

vivekasopānaparamparāṇām // [84]

Having risen higher and higher the intellect will see without being aware of any fatigue the highest truth which happened to be the result of the intellectual heritage formulated by our predecessors.

The text consists of four *khaṇḍas*. The first *khaṇḍa* consists of sixteen sub-chapters named *adhyāyas*. In the first *adhyāya* named *ayuṣkāmīyakalpa* the origin of Āyurveda, ten types of sins leading to various diseases, daily routine etc are mentioned in forty-three *kārikas* (verses).

An example from this portion is cited below to illustrate the interrelation between *Aṣṭāṅgahṛdaya* and *Hṛdayapriya.*

brāhme muhūrte uttiṣṭhet

svastho rakṣārthamāyuṣaḥ /

śarīracintām nirvartya

kṛtaśaucavidhistataḥ // [85]

brāhme muhūrte uttiṣṭhet

āyuśrīsukhavṛddhaye //

kṛtaśaucaḥ smarennityam

ihāmutra ca yacchubham // [86]

In the second chapter named *śālyādikalpa,* the qualities of coconut water, milk, coconut oil etc are explained. The qualities of the coconut oil is described here thus:

nāḷikerodbhavam tailam

bṛhaṇam balavardhanam /

vṛṣyam tridoṣaśamanam

madhuram dantarogajit // [87]

The oil produced out of coconut increases energy, and sexual potency maintains the equilibrium of tridoṣas, and prevents dental diseases.

In the third chapter named *dravyajñānakalpa* qualities of the different medicinal materials are mentioned in six *vargas* (categories). In the fourth chapter named *āhārādikalpa* unnecessary suppression of the natural urges and the diseases coming out of that and qualities of the meat as food are mentioned. In the fifth chapter named *rasādinirūpaṇakalpa,* different types of rasas and qualities, etc; are mentioned. In the sixth chapter named *garbhopacārakalpa* the treatment of pregnancy, disorders of pregnancy and their remedies are described. In the seventh chapter named *bālarogapratiṣedhakalpa* the disease common to children and their treatment are described. In the eighth chapter named *aṅgavijñānakalpa,* the *pañcabhūta* elements in the body and the organs of the body are mentioned. In the ninth chapter named *snehasvedakalpa* different types of medicinal oils and their application are described. In the tenth chapter named *vamanavirecanakalpa* the eradication of diseases through womitting and purgation are described in detail. In the eleventh chapter named *vastikalpa* three types of *vasti* and the procedures followed to do *vasti* are explained in detail. In twelfth chapter named *nasyādikalpa* the three types of *nasya* and the treatment of diseases of the eyes and nose are described in detail. In the 13th chapter named *raktamokṣakalpa* the qualities of pure blood, impure blood and the expulsion of the impure blood, etc; are mentioned. In the 14th chapter named *kṣārāgnikalpa* the qualities of the *kṣāra* (ashes) and their proper usage in various treatment (causterisation), etc.; are mentioned. In the fifteenth chapter named *yantraśastrādikalpa* the manufacturing methods of different *yantras* (machines) for *vasti, dhūmanāli* (catheter), etc; are explained in detail In the sixteenth chapter named *dravyādikalpa* description of the place from where medicinal materials are to be collected and the classification of medicinal herbs are given in detail.

The second *khaṇḍa* consists of eighteen sub-chapters. In the first *adhyāya* named *dūtalakṣaṇādhyāya* the description of the qualities of a *dūta* (messenger) and the condition of the disease of the patient conveyed by his from the mere appearance are explained. In the second chapter named *jvaracikitsādhyāya* the different types of fever and their treatments are given. In the third chapter named *raktapittādicikitsādhyāya* different types of *raktapitta* (bleeding) and their treatments are mentioned. It is interesting to note that in this chapter *gaṇeśapūjā* (worship of Lord Ganapati) is also recommended as a complementary treatment for *raktapitta*.

> *nityam raktaprasāntyartham*
>
> *gaṇeśam ca prapūjayet //* [88]

For obtaining cure from *raktapitta*, Lord Gaṇeśa should be worshipped daily.

In the fourth chapter named *śvāsahidhmācikitsitam* different types of respiratory diseases and their treatments are mentioned. In the fifth chapter named *rajayakṣmāsvarasādārocakacikitsā,* the treatment for *rājayakṣmā* (Tuberculosis) is described in detail. In the sixth chapter named *charddihṛdrogatṛṣṇācikitsitam*, different types of emesis and heart diseases and their treatments are given. In the seventh chapter named *madātyayarśaudavartacikitsitam;* different types of mental disorders and abdominal diseases and their treatment are explained. In the eighth chapter named *astisāragrahaṇyatyagnicikitsitam,* diarrhea, intense hunger, etc; and their treatments are given. In the ninth chapter named *mūtrakṛcchacikitsitam* different types of urinary diseases and their treatment are mentioned. In the tenth chapter named *pramehanidānam* twenty types of diabetes and their treatment are explained. In the eleventh chapter named *vidradhivṛddhicikitsita* different types of *vidradhi* (ulcers), *vṛddhi* (cancers) and their treatments are explained. In the twelfth chapter *gulmacikitsitam* eight types of *gulma* (abdominal tumours) and their treatments are explained. In the thirteenth chapter named *pāṇḍuśophacikitsitam* different types of skin diseases and their treatment are explained. In the fourteenth chapter named *udaracikitsita* different types of abdominal diseases and their treatment are explained. In the fifteenth chapter named *visarpamasūrikavisphoṭasitāpittakusṭhacikitsitam* the treatment of *masūri* (small pox) fever, leprosy, etc; are given in detail. In the sixteenth chapter named *śvitrakṣudrakṛmicikitsita* the treatment of leucoderma (a type of skin disease) diseases caused by worms parasite inside the abdomen), etc; are mentioned. In the seventeenth chapter named *vātacikitsā* different types of gouts and their treatment are explained. In the eighteenth chapter named *raktavātavraṇabhaṅgacikitsā* the treatment for *raktavāta*, different types of ulcers coming out of various gouts are described in detail.

The third *khaṇḍa* consists of fourteen sub-chapters. The first chapter, named as *śirorogacikitsita*, gives cures for the diseases above the neck and their treatments in detail. In the second chapter named *vartmarogacikitsita* the cause for *vartma disease* (diseases of eyelids) and their treatment are explained in detail. In the third chapter named *sandhisitāsitacikitsita* cause and treatment for different types of diseases in the joints are explained in detail. In the fourth chapter named *dṛṣṭirogacikitsita* the cause of various diseases in the eye and their treatments are explained in detail.

In the fifth chapter named *sarvākṣirogacikitsita* the treatment of all other diseases in the eye other than those mentioned in the fourth chapter, is described in detail. In the sixth chapter named *nāsārogacikitsitam* the diseases of the nose and their treatments are explained in detail. In seventh chapter named *karṇarogacikitsita* the causes and treatments of various diseases of ears are mentioned. In the eighth chapter named *mukharogacikitsita* the causes and treatment of various oral diseases are mentioned. In the ninth chapter named *gaṇḍamālānālīvraṇādicikitsita* causes and cures of various diseases of the neck are described. In the tenth chapter named *guhyarogacikitsā* various disease of the genital organsand their treatments are described. In the eleventh chapter named *bhagandaraślīpadacikitsita* various diseases of the rectum and their treatments are mentioned. In the twelfth chapter named *viṣacikitsitam* various types of diseases of snake-bit, etc; and their treatments are mentioned. In the thirteenth chapter named *rasāyanavidhāna* the qualities of *rasāyana* elixir and their preparations are explained. In the fourteenth chapter named *vajīkaraṇam* different types of *vajīkaraṇa* (Virilification therapy) are explained.

The fourth *khaṇḍa* is named as *yogakhaṇḍa*. This *khaṇḍa* consists of twelve sub-chapters, giving details about different types of *yogas* (recipes) for the preparation of medicine. This *khaṇḍa*concludes with the verse thus:

evam sthānatraye 'pyādidevena grathitāstu ye

yogāste 'pi kramāt proktāḥ santastuṣyantu santatam iti / [89]

Thus all the *yogas* (recipes) composed by *ādideva* (Brahmā) are described in order by me in the three chapters are already described here one by one. The scholars may be pleased by this.

It is remarkable to note that Vaikkam Pāccumūttatu gives the causes (*nidāna*) and treatment (*cikitsā*) at the same place, which would be very useful to the Āyurvedic physicians. Most of the medicines prescribed in this text have been widely using by the Āyurvedic scholars of Kerla.

F. *SUKHASĀDHAKA*

It is a short treatise on Āyurveda composed with the aim of treating the common diseases which prevailed during Pāccumūttatu's time and the medicine used by himself to eradicate them. This can be inferred from the *śloka* (verse) at the end of the text named *avasiṣṭa*.

Itisarvacikitsoktā samkṣepātsiddhabheṣajaiḥ. / [90]

The only treatments adopted me and proved successful in my own experience are given here.

The text consists of twelve *khaṇḍas*. The first *khaṇḍaa* consists of four sub chapters named *sāmānyādhikāra*, *jvarādhikāra*, *sannipātalakṣaṇa* and *sannipātacikitsā*. The first chapter *sāmānyādhikāra* begins with the *maṅgaḷaśloka* (benedictory verse) thus :

namo nārāyaṇāyastu

gurave karuṇātmane /

āyurvedopadeśena

sarveṣām sukhadāyine // [91]

I offer my salutations to lord Nārāyaṇa the preceptor, of Āyurveda, on whose grace depends the well being of the whole universe.

In this portion a brief account of the topic going to be presented is given. In the second chapter named *jvarādhikāra* different types of fever and their treatments are given. In the third and fourth portion named *sannipātalakṣaṇa* and *sannipātacikitsā* the causes and treatment of *sannipāta* are described.

The second khaṇḍa consists of twelve sub-chapters. They are raktapittādhikāra, pradarādhikāra, asthisravādhikāra, kāsādhikara, śvāsādhikāra, rājayakṣmādhikāra, svarasādhikāra, arocakādhikāra, hṛdrogādhikāra, tṛṣṇādhikāra, charddyadhikāra, madamūrchā sanyadhikāra. This khaṇḍa consists of the description of different types of respiratory diseaes, tuberculosis, heart disease, vomiting etc and their treatments. The third khaṇḍa combined of six sub-chapters. They are arśodhikāra, udavartādhikāra, atisārādhikāra, grahaṇyadhikāra, viṣūcikādhikāra and atyagnyadhikāra. In this khaṇḍa various diseases of the rectum, diarrhea, etc and their treatments are given. The fourth khaṇḍa consists of of three sub-chapters. They are mūtrakṛcchādhikāra, pramehādhikāra and piṭakādhikāra. In this khaṇḍa different types of urinary disorders, diabetes and their treatments are explained pañcamakhaṇḍa consists of five subchapters. They are pāṇḍvadadhikāra, śophādhikāra, vṛddhyadhikāra, gunmādhikāra, mahodarādhikāra. This khaṇḍa deals with different types of skin disease, gas trouble, and other diseases of the abdomen and their treatments in detail. Ṣaṣthakhaṇḍa consists of five subchapters. They are visarpādhikāra, masūrikādhikāra, kuṣṭhādhikāra, śvitrādhikāra and kṛmirogādhikāra. This khaṇḍa deals with leprocy, masūri (small pox), (leucoderma) etc and their treatment in detail.The saptamakhaṇḍa consists of three sub-chapters. They are vātavyādhyadhikāra, vātaśoṇitādhikāra and vraṇādhikāra. This khaṇḍa deals with different types of rheumatic diseases and the ulcers arising from it and their treatment in detail.

The eighth *khaṇḍa* consists of six sub-chapters. They are *śirorogādhikāra, netracikitsā, sitāsitarogādhikāra, dṛṣṭirogādhikāra and sarvākṣirogādhikāra.* This *khaṇḍa* deals with the diseases above neck, especially eyes in detail with their effective treatment.

The ninth *khaṇḍa* consists of three sub-chapters. They are *karṇarogādhikāra, nāsārogādhikāra, āsyarogādhikāra.* This *khaṇḍa* deals with the diseases of the ear, nose and mouth and their medicines in detail.

The tenth *khaṇḍa* consists of four sub-chapters. They are *gaṇḍarogādhikāra, guhyarogādhikāra, bhagandaraślīpadādhikāra* and *kṣudrarogādhikāra.* This *khaṇḍa* deals with various disease of the neck, diseases of the genital organs, piles and their treatments.

The eleventh *khaṇḍa* contains of five chapters called *sarpaviṣādhikāra, kīṭādiviṣādhikāra, lūtādiviṣādhikāra, ākhuviṣādhikāra and damṣṭriviṣādhikāra* respectively. This deals with different types of toxin by the biting of the snakes, spider and other little creatures and their medicines.

The twelfth *khaṇḍa* consists of three subchapters. They are *garbhādhikāra, bālopacārādhikāra and avaśiṣṭam.* This *khaṇḍa* consist of treatment of pregnancy and childhood. The last chapter *avaśiṣṭa* is the conclusion of the subject mentioned in the text. The text ends with the *śloka*:

> *Śivadvijena bhiṣajā dhiyā 'dāyākalīdṛśaḥ*
>
> *grantaḥ kenāpyanyatantrāt rogiṇām sukhasādhakaḥ //* [92]

This text is composed by a *Śivadvija* collecting material from other medicinal texts for the well being of the patients.

The word *bhiṣaja dhiyā 'dāya* is the Kali date of the completion of the text; the Malayalam era is equal to 1057 ciṅṅa – 22 (1882AD)

This text seems to be planned as a hand book, which serves a ready reference for physicians in their treatment of the common diseases like fever, etc.

Other Works

Vaikkam Pāccumūttatu's known other non-Āyurvedic works are:

1) *Rāmavarmacarita* – a poem in eight cantos on Āyilyam Tirunāḷ Mahārāja of Travancore.

2) *Nakṣatramālā*

3) *Kāśiyātrā*

4) *Sukhasādhaka*

5) *Sukhabodhika*

6) *Arthavimarśinī* commentary on *Rājasūyaprabandha* of Melputtūr Nārāyaṇabhaṭṭa.

Malayalam Works

1) *Mucukundamokṣam* – this belongs to Āṭṭakkathā cetegory of fine Arts.

2) *Kāśiyātrāvarṇanam Oṭṭan tuḷḷal* – This work belongs to a particular Kerala fine arts propagated by Kuñjan Nambiar.

3) *Bālabhūṣaṇam*

4) *Malayāḷabhāṣāvyākaraṇam*

5) *Keralavieṣamāhātmyam.*

Another work of the author deserves special mention is *Tiruvitāṅkūr Caritram*. It is the first history of Travancore written in Malayalam. Dr.Rajan Gurukkal and Dr.Raghava Varrier in their *Keralacaritram* pays high regard to Vaikkam

Pāccumūttatu. They quoted a passage from Vaikkam Pāccumūttatu's work to substantiate his authority.

valiya āḷinte svabhāvatteyum jīvitattil ceytirikunna upakāraṅṅaḷeyum bhūmi mutalāya sampādyatteyum mattu guṇaṅṅaḷeyum uddeśiccu satyamāyittuḷḷa vacanavistāramākunnu. [93]

'The history should be the true record of the following'.

1)   The character and deeds of a reputed individual,

2)   The service or contribution done by that individual to society

3)   Details about his wealth, including possession of land, etc.)

They pointed out that this is the new approach in the field of history.[94]

G. *DHĀRĀKALPA*

Dhārākalpa is the only available text on *dhārācikitsā*, which is considered to be an original contribution of Kerala to Āyurveda. This work is written by Āttupuratt Impiccan Gurukkal.[95] Born at Koyilandy in Kozhikide district as the son of Āttupuratt Chathu and Cettiyedath Coyichi in the year 1852, Impiccan Gurukkal studied Sanskrit language under Uppoṭṭ Kaṇṇan when reading the proof of the commentary on *Aṣṭāṅgahṛdaya* by the latter. Ullūr pointed out that 'Gurukkal' may be the surname used by the teachers belonging to castes like Kaṇiśa, Kammāla and Tiyya in North Malabar.[96] This work seems to be a collection of methods of treatment prevailing in Kerala before the advent of Sanskrit *Samhitā* texts on Āyurveda.

Dhārākalpa is a short treatise on Āyurveda which deals with different types of *dhārā* treatment prevailed only in Kerala. The text is available at the end of *Sahasrayoga* text published from Kerala. North Indian version of *Sahasrayoga* does not contain this portion. The author begins the work, paying homage to Lord Gaṇeśa thus:

anantakalyāṇaguṇaikabhājanam

nirantarānanda cidekavigraham /

anantarāyepsitasiddhaye vayam

tamekadantam satatam bhajāmahe // [97]

In order to accomblish our desired end with out obstacles we offer prayers to Lord Gaṇēśa who has one tusk, who is the abode of infinite good qualities, infinite blessings, and who possess a body which is the combination of continuous bliss and consciousness.

The text consists of thirty four verses (*kārikas*). With these thirty four *kārikas* he has enumerated the *dhārācikitsā* very effectively. This proves his poetic talent, brevity and mastery over Sanskrit language.

After the salutation to *iṣṭadevatā*, the author explains the qualities of *dhārā* treatment. Thus:

> *dhātūnām dṛḍhatām karoti vṛṣatām dehāgnivarṇaujasām*
>
> *sthairyam pāṭavamindriyasya jarasomāndyam ciram jīvitam /*
>
> *asthnāmbhaṅgamapākaroti nitarām doṣān samīrādikān*
>
> *sarvasnehakṛtā sukheṣṇasubhagā sarvāṅgadhārā nṛṇām //* [98]

Dhārā treatment improves physical strength, sexual potency, good apetite and good colour. It also strengthens the constituent elements of the body, strengthens the bones, removes the old age problems and provides good health and longevity to the human beings.

In the following verses the author gives a list of trees that are suitable for making the *dhārā* vessel. It is interesting to note that *dhārā* vessel is commonly seen in rich families of Kerala. Nowadays and it is generally called as *dhārāpātti* and the treatment is known as *pātticikitsā*. (see the illustrations at the end)

The trees recommended for the making of *dhārā* vessel is given thus:

> *plakṣodumbara gandhasāra varaṇa nyagrodha devadrumāḥ*
>
> *punāgāhva kapitha coca bakuḷāśokāsanāmrastathā /*
>
> *doḷā campaka vilvanimbakhadirāmoghāgnimanthārjjunāḥ*
>
> *ityādyanyatamena secanavidhau droṇīm prakuryāt budhāḥ //* [99]

The dhārā vessel should be made out of any one of these trees by a vaidya: itti (Ficus Microcorpa), atti (Gularfig), candanam (Sandal wood) nīrmātaḷam (Three leaved caper), perāl (Banyan) devatāram (Deodar) punna (Alexander laurel) vilārmaram (Elephant apple)] vayaṇa (Cinnamon) ilaññi (Bullet tree wood) aśoka (Ashoka) veṅṅa (Indian kino tree) māv (mango tree) ḍolimaram or koli (Flowering muda), campakam (champak) kūvaḷam (Holy fruit tree) vep (Nimba) kariṅṅāli (Cutch tree), pātiri (Yellow snake tree) muñña (Premna corymbosa) nīrmarut (Arjun)

In the next verse the author gives the measurement for the preparation of *dhārā* vessel thus:

droṇīhastacatuṣkadīrghakaramātra vyāsatatpādamā-

trodyatbhittiyutādṛḍhā samatalā pādāntarandhrābahiḥ /

śīrṣasthāna ihonnataika karamātrātānavistārakā

nimnā kiñcanamaddhyataśca caraṇairhastaiścayuktā dṛḍhaiḥ // [100]

The length and breadth of the *dhārā* vessel should be in the ratio 4:1 *hasta*[101] and height of the sides is six *aṅgulas*.[102] Moreover inner surface of the vessel should be softened and concaved. It should have a hole at the leg portion. The head portion is slightly higher than leg portion and the vessel should be supported by strong hand and legs.

Small vessels required for *dhārā* treatment are also mentioned here. Small vessels should be made out of gold, silver or mud. The method of preparation of mud pot for this purpose is also explained in detail. In the following verses the qualities required for the assistants (nurses) and the procedures of the treatment are explained thus:

grāhyāste paricārakāsyuraunuraktāssāvadhānaśśubhā –

yetaddhassudṛḍhāvalambanavaśāttalpātrapātāditiḥ /

bhītirjātu cidāturasya tu yathā nasyattatha kāraye-

ddhārām mūrddhani hastayorapi pṛthagvakṣaḥsthale pādayoḥ // [103]

Those persons who are compassionate who are vigilant and who are endowed with good conduct should be selected as nurses. The patient should have faith in the nurses to believe that the pots held high would not fall down from their hands. *dhārā* treatment should be done simultaneously on head, both hands and both legs.

In the next verses the author explained the procedures of *śirovasti* and the advantages of applying oil to hair during *dhārā* treatment. After that the good results obtained by *dhārā* treatment using buttermilk is explained as follows:

keśādīnāñca śaukḷyam kḷamamapitanutām doṣakopam śirorug

bādhāmojaḥkṣayam talkaracaraṇaparistodanam mūtradoṣam /

sandhīnām viślathatvam hṛdayarugarucī jātharāgneśca māndyam

dhātrītakrothadhārā haratiśirasivā karṇanetrāmayaugham // [104]

The *dhārā* treatment with the juice of *āmalakī* (Emblic myrobalan) and buttermilk prevents whitening of hairs, increases physical strength (energy), cures headache, urinary diseases, heart diseases, increases appetite and prevents diseases of the ears and eyes.

After explaining the procedures of different *dhārā* treatment, in detail, the author warns about the diseases and their remedies coming out of improper procedures followed during treatment. If the level of the pot from which medicine is poured on the fore-head is not proper, it leads to vomiting, fever, skin diseases and other diseases. Remedies like gargling with medicine, (*gaṇḍūṣa*) using of nasal medicine (*nasya*) and the intake of dried ginger are recommended.

The text ends with the list of restrictions that should be observsed by the patient under treatment thus:

vyāyāmātapavegarodhahimadhūmatyuccanīcopadhā —

nāhaḥ svapnarajaḥ pravātacirakālāsīnatāsamsthitiḥ /

śokam jāgarapādayānagamanakrodhādi bhāṣyādikān

styaktva 'thoṣṇajalopacāryanatibhuksyātbrahmacārī sadā // [105]

During the treatment one should abstain from doing hard work, exposure to sunlight, smoke or fog etc, unwanted control over natural urges, standing or sitting at a place for a long time, travelling for a long time, sleeping during day time, and waking during night time. It is advisable to use hot water for bath and observe celebacy etc. also.

It deserves special mention to note that *Dhārākalpa* forms the basis of the treatment called *sukhacikitsā,* prevaling in Kerala which has been attracting foreigners to here.

Non-Āyurvedic works

The author's other works include a Sanskrit poem named *Raghavāmṛta,* Sanskrit commentary on *Manīṣāpañcaka* of Śaṅkarācārya, A commentary in Malayalam on *Praveśaka,* by Tṛkkaṇḍiyūr Acyutapiṣāroṭi and Translation of *Kathāsaritsāgara.*

H. *ĀROGYAKALPADRUMA*

It is a short treatise on *bālacikitsā* (paediatrics) by Kaikkuḷaṅṅara Rāma Vārrier. Kaikkuḷaṅṅara Rāma Vārrier was one of the most outstanding scholars of his time. He was born at Kaikkuḷaṅṅara Kizhakke Vāriam in Talappiḷḷi Taluk, as the son of Nārāyaṇi Vārasyār and Kaitakkoṭṭ Bhaṭṭatiri on 1883.[106] He was educated at home by his uncles Rāma Vārrier and Kṛṣṇa Vārrier, masters in *vaidya* and *jyotiṣa* respectively. He got his higher education in Vyākaraṇa, Alaṅkāra and Tarka from Govindan Nambiar of Pālappurattu Putiyeṭam. After that he studied advanced texts on Tarka from Bhīmācārya and Vedānta from Yogānanda Svāmikaḷ at Mayippadi in South Canara. Yogānanda conferred on him three titles *vāgdāsa rāmānandanātha* and *paṇḍitapārasavendra*. [107] For some time he lived at Punnattur Palace, teaching the princes there. Later he worked at Kunnamkulam and Trissur and wrote many books in Sanskrit and Malayalam.

Works

About thirty works are known to his credit. Among these works *Ārogyakalpadruma* deserves special mention because it is a compilation of the medicines prevailed among the common folks of Kerala.

Ārogyakalpadruma — An Overview

Ārogyakalpadruma[108] is a compilation of special preparations of medicine which prevailed at that time among the *Vaidyas* (Physicians) of Kerala. This can be inferred from the opening verse of this text thus:

> *atha bālacikitsaiṣā vṛddhavaidyamatānugā*
>
> *mandabuddyupakārāya pṛthageva vitanyate //* [109]

Bālacikitsā (Paediatry) followed by experts in that field, is separately dealt with here for the benefit of people of modest intelligence.

The text consists of fourty chapters. The treatment of the child upto sixteen years is mentioned in it. Bāla is defined as the child up to sixteen years. In the first *adhyāya* (chapter) the treatment of the child upto fifteen days after birth is explained in detail. The products of coconut are widely recommended as ingredients for medicines in this work. Coconut milk is recommended as hair oil for infants in this chapter thus:

> *svasthasya pratyaham snānam*
>
> *hitamabhyaṅgapūrvakam /*
>
> *abhyaṅge nāḷikerasya*
>
> *payaḥ kevalamiṣyate //* [110]

Healthy infant should be bathed daily after gentle massage only with coconut milk.

This seems to be a practice prevalent in Kerala *gṛhavaidya* which exists nowadays also.

In the second chapter the treatment of the infants after fifteen days and the methods of the removal of impurities (*doṣas*) in mothers milk are described in detail.

In the third chapter named *jvaracikitsādhyāya* various types of fever and their treatment are explained in detail. It is interesting here to note that some bizarre medicines are also recommended:

> *makkuṇān gulasanchannān*
>
> *bhakṣayedvā yathārhataḥ /*
>
> *cāturthikajvare vaidyo*
>
> *rahasyamidamauṣadham //* [111]

Bugs covered in jaggery are recommended as medicine for fever which repeats every four days (*cāturthikajvara*). This is also mentioned as a secret medicine.

The fourth chapter consists of three sub-divisions. In the first sub division named *raktapittacikitsā* medicines for diseases connected with different types of bleeding from nose, eyes etc are described in detail. In the second portion named *kāsacikitsā* different type of cough diseases connected with lungs and their medicines are mentioned. In the fifth chapter named *kṣayacikitsā* different types of medicines for *kṣaya* (tuberculosis) are described. The remedy recommended here for the disease caused by over consumption of tobacco makes interesting reading.

> *nāḷikeraphalakṣīre,*
>
> *katakasya rajaḥ pibet /*
>
> *śāntaye dhūpapatro 'tha*
>
> *vikārāṇām thatā sitām //* [112]

In take of *kaṭaka* (water cleaning seed) powder in coconut milk or coconut milk mixed with sugar solution, will cure the ailments caused by over consumption of tobacco.

The sixth chapter consists of four portions. The first portion named as *arśacikitsā* contains description of various types of piles and their medicines. The second portion named *grahaṇicikitsā* containsdiscription of various types of *grahaṇis* (dysentry) and their medicines. The third portion named *kṛmicikitsā*, contains various kinds of medicines for the diseases caused by worms. The seventh chapter consists of two portions. The first portion called as *mūtrāghātacikitsā*, describes different types of urinary diseases and their remedies.

In the second portion named as *piṭakacikitsā* the medicines recommended for different types of scabies and herpes are explained in detail.

The eighth chapter consists of five portions. The first portion called as *vṛddhicikitsā* consists of remedies for different types of *vṛddhis* (enlargement) of the scrotum etc; The second portion named as *gunmacikitsā* consists of remedies for various types of *gunma* (abdominal tumour). The third portion named as *mahodaracikitsā* contains the remedies for *mahodara* (enlargement of abdomen) especially in the elders.

The fourth portion named as *pāṇḍucikitsā* consists of various medicines for *pāṇḍu* (anaemia) The fifth portion named as *kāmilācikitsā* contains different types of medicines for *kāmila* (jaundice.) In the Ninth chapter named *visarpanidāna* detailed descriptions of nine types of *visarpas* (a kind of skin disease) are given. In the tenth chapter the treatments of the skin diseases (*visarpa or karappan*) are given. The *visarpa* disease seen in children is called *karappan*. It is interesting here to note that the medicine recommended for *karappan* contains coconut milk as an ingredient as follows:

> *piṣṭvā gopātmajāmūlam*
>
> *parṇavatyāstvajo 'pi va /*
>
> *kṣīreṇa nāḷikerasya*
>
> *limpedatra muhurmuhuḥ //* [113]

Grind the root of *naruniṇḍi* (country sarasaparilla) or vembālapaṭṭa (bark of devil tree) and mix it with coconut milk and apply it to the affected parts again and again.

Also

> *śatāhvām nāḷikerasya*
>
> *piṣṭvā kṣīreṇa lepayet /*
>
> *dhānyakaḥ praśamam yāti*
>
> *tanmātreṇa navotthitaḥ //* [114]

Grind *śatakuppa* (Dill) in coconut milk and apply the affected parts it will cure the newly formed *dhānyaka* (a type of *karappan*).

In the eleventh, twelfth and thirteen chapters detailed descriptions of *karappans* like *black gram karappan*, (elkarappan), *thorn karappan (mulkarappan)s* and their medicines are found. It is remarkable that most of the medicines recommended contains coconut milk as an ingredient. The medicine recommended for *blackgram karappan* is given here to illustrate the above point:

> *payasā nāḷikerasya*
>
> *pārantīmulavatkalā //* [115]

Grind the root of tetti (jungle-flame ixora) in coconut milk and apply it the affected parts.

The fourteenth chapter is devoted to the treatment of *visarpa* (herps) named as *visarpasāmānyacikitsā*.

The fifteenth chapter is named as *masūrilakṣaṇa* (small pox). It contains detailed description of *masūri* diseases and its effective treatments. This treatment also uses coconut milk as an ingredient as follows:

> *nāḷikerasya dugdhena*
>
> *piṣṭvā candanagairike /*
>
> *amṛtacandanośira-*
>
> *nyathavātra tu lepanam //* [116]

Apply coconut milk mixed with sandal and red soil or apply coconut milk mixed with *amṛta*, sandal and *rāmacca.* (vetiver)

The sixteenth chapter called *kuṣṭhacikitsā* contains the description of various types of leprosy with effective treatment and named as *kuṣṭhacikitsā*. The seventeenth chapter named as *vātavyādhicikitsā* contains treatment of various types of gouts.   The eighteenth chapter named as *raktastambhanidāna* contains the causes and effective treatment of diseases caused by impure blood.

The ninteenth chapter named as *kuṇḍalakalakṣaṇa* contains the causes and effective treatment of bulging in human body. The twentieth chapter named as *śākharogalakṣaṇa* contains the description and effective treatment of the diseases of the hands and legs. The twenty-first chapter is named *nābhīrogacikitsanam*. It contains the treatments of diseases in the exterior parts of a body like umbilical region.

The twenty-second chapter is named as *vraṇacikitsakaḷ*. It contains different types of bruises and scabies at different part of human body with effective treatment.

The twenty-third chapter named as *bhagandaracikitsā* contains detailed description of diseases of the rectum with effective treatment.

The twentyfifth chapter named as *liṅgavyādhicikitsā*, contains details about various types of diseases connected with genital organs with their effective treatment.

The twenty-sixth chapter is devoted to the treatment of the diseases of the eyes and is named as *netrarogacikitsā*. *Netrāmṛtam* of Vallathol seems to be the translation of the above work because Vallathol translated *Ārogyakalpadruma* and gave a new name to it as *Ārogyacintāmaṇi*. However nothing definite can be said about this matter because *Netrāmṛtam* and *netrarogacikitsā* by the author are not available now. It is particular here to note that in the beginning of this portion the author declared that he is going to deal this portion in a separate text so a brief account of it only given here.[117] The preparation of *Ilanīrkuzhampu* which is an ideal Kerala medicine prepared out of tender coconut is mentioned.[118]

The twenty-seventh chapter deals with the treatment of the diseases connected with ears and is named as *karṇarogacikitsā*. The twenty-eighth chapter deals with the treatment of the diseases connected with nasal organs named as *nāsārogacikitsā*. The twenty-ninth chapter describes various diseases of the mouth with effective treatment and is named as *mukharogacikitsā*. The thirtieth chapter deals with treatment of the diseases of the head with effective treatment and is named as *śirorogacikitsā*. The thirty-first chapter is devoted to various psychological diseases with effective treatment and is named as *unmādacikitsā*. The thirty-second chapter deals with epilepsy and its treatment and is named as *apasmārarogacikitsā*. The thirty-third chapter deals with the protection of children from evil spirits deities responsible for diseases and is named as *bālagrahopadravapratividhi*. The thirty-fourth chapter deals with the causes and effective treatment of the diseases caused by a graha named Śakuni. So it is named as *pakṣipīḍālakṣaṇacikitsā*. The thirty-fifth chapter gives the list of medicines which are helpful to increase the immunity power of the newly born up to twelve years; it is named as *prakārayogas*. The thirty-sixth chapter deals with the toxicology and is named as *viṣādicikitsā*. The thirty-seventh chapter deals with the medicines that should be consumed to cure ailments caused by over consumption of the food items. It is interesting here to note that the medicines prescribed here are entirely different from the medicines for the same purpose in *Sahasrayoga.*The thirty-eighth chapter deals with the purification process of the various medicinal raw materials. The thirty-ninth chapter deals with the treatment of the man and woman separately. It is named as *pariśiṣṭacikitsāprayogas.*

The text ends with the fortieth chapter which deals with measures to be taken after seeing the head of the child during childbirth. Kaikkuḷaṅṅara Rāma Vārrier at the concluding portion proclaimes that though the text contains treaments meant for children up to 16 years the medicines are useful for grown ups too. Further he wishes that let his work might be accepted by all.[119]

Other works

Kaikkuḷaṅṅara Rāma Vārrier's other works include several commentaries on Sanskrit and Malayalam. His important Malayalam commentaries include commentaries on the following Sanskrit works.

(1)	*Raghuvamśa*	(2)	*Māgha*
(3)	*Naiṣadha*	(4)	*Kumārasambhava*
(5)	*Meghasandeśa*	(6)	*Yuthiṣṭhiravijaya*
(7)	*Kṛṣṇavilāsa*	(7)	*Bhāvaprakāśavyākhyā* on *Aṣṭāṅgahṛdaya*, which is a beautiful commentary on *Aṣṭāṅgahṛdaya* in lucid style even understandable to common man.
(8)	*Amarakośa*	(9)	*Siddhāntakaumudī* (pūrvārdha)
(10)	*Horā*	(11)	*Praśnatraya*
(12)	*Amarukaśataka*	(13)	*Devīsaptaśati*
(14)	*Gītagovinda* and	(15)	*Mahiṣamaṅgalam Bhāṇa.*

In Sanskrit he wrote commentary called *preyasī* on three cantos of *Kumārasambhava*. His original works in Sanskrit consist of the *stotras: Vagānāndalaharī* in praise of the Goddess of speech in 108 verses written in *śikhariṇī* metre on the model of Śaṅkara's *Saundaryalaharī, Vāmadevastava* in Sragdharā metre praising god Siva, *Vidyunmālāstuti* and *Vidyākṣaramālā*. He himself wrote the *Hṛdya* commentary on *Vāgānandalaharī* and the *Arthaprakāśikā* commentary on the *Vāmadevastava.*[120]

I. *Aṣṭāṅgaśarīra*

It an important work on *Āyurveda* composed by Vaidyaratnam P.S Varrier. The contribution of P.S Varrier to the field of *Āyurveda* deserves special mention because he had lifted Āyurveda from its traditional inert state of stagnation and made it relevant to the contemporary society. He not only composed works like *Aṣṭāṅgaśarīra* and *Bṛhacchārīra* on *Āyurveda* by incorporating principles from allopathic systems but also established institutions like *pāṭhaśālas* and *āryavaidyaśālā*. He also propagated Āyurveda through a magazine called *Dhanvantarī*. It can be stated that if the present day world knows about the unique Āyurvedic tradition of kerala, it is largely due to the yeoman service done by P.S.Vārrier.

The Date of the Author and Personal Details

P. S Varrier was born on 16th March of 1869 A.D corresponding to the Malayalam Era 4th Mīnam of 1044. From the introductory verse of the *Bṛhacchārīra* it can be gathered that his father was Rāma Vārrier of Māṅkuḷaṅṅara Vāriem and mother was Kunhikutty vārasyār (Śrīpārvati) of Pannīnpalli vārriem.

> *Vikhyāto 'jani rāmapārśvajavaro mṛdvāpikūlālaye*
>
> *Preyasyāsyā varāhacaityasadane śrīpārvatī cābhavat /*
>
> *Dampatyoranayorupāttatapasoḥ putraḥ pavitrātmanoḥ*
>
> *spaṭārtham racayāmi samprati bṛhacchārīramārṣāspadam //*[121]

Son of the famous Māṅkuḷaṅṅara Rāma Vārrier and Pannīnpalli Śrīpārvati, the couple who acquired the merit of penance and who were endowed with pure thoughts, I am composing this *Bṛhacchārīra* on the basis of the utterings of the sages with a view to elucidating their teachings.

P.S Varrier's grandfather Śaṅkaran was a great Āyurvedic physician of that time. So the parents gave the very name to the grandson P.S Varrier started his education at the age of four under his uncle Kuṭṭikṛṣṇa Vārrier and taught him learned Sanskrit language under various eminent scholars.[122] He studied preliminary lessons of *Āyurveda* from Konoth Acyutavārier who was a disciple of Kuṭṭañjeri Mūsad. Then he studied under Kuṭṭañjeri Vāsudevan Mūsad, one of the famous *aṣṭavaidyas* of that time and started practicing at Koṭṭakkal.

P.S Varrier studied the principles of allopathic system under Dr. Varghese who was a surgeon in the government hospital. He had approached Dr. Varghese for a minor eye operation and this contact developed into close friendship and P.S Varrier studied modern anatomy and physiology from him. Later on he incorporated this modern knowledge also into the works composed by him on *Āyurveda*.

Although P.S Varrier was deeply religious and traditional in beliefs and practices his attitude towards other faiths was influenced by cosmopolitan principles. Dr. K.N Panickar observes thus; P.S Varrier was free from many of the prejudices of his time. Varrier had an open critical and eclectic mind'.[123] The broad vision and realistic attitude of P.S Varrier towards *Āyurveda* can be inferred from the passage of *Dhanvantarī* from the following words :

The antiquity of *Āyurveda* is a matter of pride for all of us, but nobody can deny that its present state is quite deplorable. Due to reasons both internal and external, our medicinal system has steadily declined while in contrast, other systems have progressed in an equal degree. The people of the West examine the laws of nature and invent new dimensions of science, thereby repeatedly reversing earlier scientific knowledge. We, on the other hand, blindly believe that old sciences are perfect. As a result, we have not only failed to progress but have also been pushed down the ladder by others. If this state of affairs continues for some more time there is no doubt that *Āyurveda* will become totally extinct. [124]

Generally P.S Varrier adopted three methods to uplift and propagate *Āyurveda*. (1) The retrieval, systematization and dissemination of knowledge. (2) Establishing institutions for giving proper training to the physicians (3) Preparation and distribution of medicines.

Varrier initiated the humble beginning of his epoch-making work with the formation of the Āryavaidyasamāja in 1902. It was essentially a voluntary public platform to exchange views and share experiences. The Mahārājas of Travancore, Cochin and Zamorin of Calicut were its patrons and P.S Varrier was nominated as its permanent secretary. The proceedings of the meetings had two sessions. The first comprised general speeches on Āyurveda aimed at to increase the confidence in the system. The second was the sharing of experiences in treatment. This helped significantly to codify the uncodified experience and innovation of different physicians. The Āryavaidyasamāja was converted into Kerala Āyurvedic studies and Research society in 1976.

In the 15th Annual meeting of Āryarvaidyasamāja on 14th January 1917 at Calicut Varrier started Pāṭhaśālā. The objective of the institution as given in the prospectus was 'to revive the once prosperous and now increasingly declining *Ayurveda*'. The emphasis had been given for mastering *Ayurveda* texts and through that acquiring knowledge of medicines and their preparations. They were supplemented with instructions in Physiology, Anatomy, Chemistry, Midwifery and Surgery adopted from Allopathy.[125] The Pāṭhaśāla was shifted to Koṭṭakkal in 1924 and later affiliated to Calicut University and renamed as Vaidyaratnam P.S Varriers Āyurveda College.

A charitable hospital named Āryavaidyacikitsāśālā was also established by Varrier on 1924. It is remarkable to note that it had a separate allopathic wing. Nowadays also as in the past this hospital provides free treatment to the patients.

The most important contribution of P.S Varrier is the establishment of Āryavaidyaśālā at Koṭṭakkal. He realised that Āyurveda treatment could be effective only if its medicines are prepared properly. So he started Āryavaidyaśālā on 12th October 1902. His progressive outlook and noble ideas are reflected in the manifesto brought out by him for Āryavaidyaśālā. In the present day also Āryavaidyaśālā is functioning according to his will. The surplus income got from Āryavaidyaśālā is earmarked for charitable purposes like the development of Āryavaidyaśālā by improving facilities, conducting seminars on Āyurveda and Research projects, providing medicines and treatment for poor patients free of cost and giving financial assistance to the Āyurveda College at Koṭṭakkal.

In recognition to the service rendered to the human society Government of India conferred him Title **Vaidyaratnam** on 1933. After 11 years in 1944 on 30th January Sunday P.S Varrier passed away.

Aṣṭāṅgaśarīra or *Laghuśarīra*-contents

It is an authoritative text on Āyurveda by P.S Varrier adopting principles and diagrams from Allopathic lore. It is meant for the students of Āyurveda so that they get acquainted with the thorough knowledge of the human body. Even though Varrier had translated many modern books on Anatomy and Physiology, unsatisfied with these efforts, Varrier composed this work with an aim to satisfy the traditional Āyurvedic scholars also. In the preface to the text Varrier quotes a *śloka* from *Carakasamhitā* and emphasises the necessity of thorough understandings of the human body runs as follows.

> *Sarvadā sarvathā sarvam*
>
> *śarīram veda yo bhiṣak /*
>
> *āyurvedam sa kārtsnyena*
>
> *veda lokasukhapradam //* [126]

That physician who knows all about the body by all means and at all times understands the Āyurveda completely for the well being of the whole world.

Varrier had coined a large number of Sanskrit words to render English terms and vice-versa while composing the text.[127] One remarkable feature of his work is the diagram of human organs with their cross-sections. Modern views about Anatomy and Physiology were rendered in beautiful Sanskrit Verses in order to enable students to memorise them easily. The text consists of 2015 verses distributed in eight chapters. The chapters are technically called as *adhyāyas*. The text begins with the benedictory verse:

> *dhanvantarīm namaskṛtya*
>
> *gurupādāmśca sādaram /*
>
> *kriyateaṣṭāṅgaśārīram*
>
> *śuddhasiddhāntagumphitam //* [128]

After saluting the God Dhanvantarī and preceptors I humbly begin to compose the work *Aṣṭāṅgaśārīra*, comprised of principles (about human body) which are made perfect by practice.

The first chapter named *garbhāvakrāntīya* consists of 164 verses. The text begins with the origin of pregnancy which runs as follows:

> *śuddhe śukḷārtave satvaḥ svakarmakleśacoditaḥ*
>
> *garbhassampadyate yuktivaśādagnirivāruṇau //* [129]

When the discharged, healthy semen is joined with ovum, pregnancy originates like fire in *araṇi*. (A stick used for producing fire for sacrificial purposes

Ideal time for marriage and progeny are given as follows:

> *tasmāt dvādaśavarṣīyamekavimśatikaḥ pumān*
>
> *udvahed vidhinā kanyāmanurūpaguṇānvitam //*

tataḥ ṣoḍaśavarṣāyām pañcavimśatikaḥ patiḥ

santatyartham yatetaiṣa kālassatputrasiddhidaḥ // [130]

Therefore a man of 21 years should marry a woman of 12 years having equal virtues and try to get a child when he attains the age of 25 years and the bride attains the age of 16 years. That is the right time for getting a heathy son.

The author warns against early attempt for begetting a child thus:

ūnaṣoḍaśavarṣāyāmaprāptaḥ pañcavimśatim

yadyādatte puman garbham kukṣisthassa vipadyate /

jāto vā na ciram jīvejjīvedvā durbalendriyaḥ // [131]

If a girl below 16 years and a man below 25 years try to get a child, the child would die in the womb itself and even if it survives the child would be weak.

The shape of the spermatozoon and ovum according to modern science are depicted in beautiful verses as follows:

pauruṣo 'yam jātamātravarṣābhūpṛthukākṛtiḥ /

śirogrīvāgātrapucchaissahitaścapalo 'niśam

yauvato guḷikākāro yalkapūrṇassabījakaḥ // [132]

The spermatozoon is like a toad of a frog with a triangular thick head, a narrow neck, a long tail and always active. The ovum is almost round in shape filled with yolk and containing a nucleus.

Then after describing the developments of the children in each month of pregnency this chapter concludes with the directions of nurturing the mother after pregnency.

The second chapter named *aṅgavibhāgādhyāya* consists of 147 verses. In this chapter different portions of the human body are decribed as follows:

śirogrīvam madhyakāyo

dvau bāhū dve ca sakthinī

ṣaḍaṅgamevamaṅgam / [133]

The head with a neck, middle portion, two upper extremities and two lower extremities; these are the six parts of the body.

Three humours called *doṣas* (*tridoṣa*) are described in this chapter thus:

vātaḥ pittam kaphaścātra

dehe doṣāstrayo matāḥ // [134]

In a human body the three humours are *vāta, pitta* and *kapha*

The functions of the veins and arteries are described as follows:

hṛdayābhimukham raktam nayantyo'tra śirā matāḥ /

tasmādbahirmukham raktam dhamanyastā vahanti yāḥ // [135]

The blood vessels which carry blood to heart are called veins (*śiraḥ*) and those which carry blood from heart are called arteries (*dhamanyaḥ*)

The five sensory organs and five motor organs are described as follows:

buddhīndriyāṇi śravaṇam sparśanam darśanam thatā

rasanam ghrāṇametāni pañca karmendriyāṇi tu

kaṇṭhapāyūpasthapāṇipādasamjñāni pañca ca // [136]

Five sensory organs are the organs of hearing, touch, sight, taste and smell. Five motor organs are the throat, rectum, genital organ, hand and foot.

In addition to the above topics this chapter deals with different layers of skin, description of cartilages etc. This chapter concludes with an advice to the aspirants who would like to lead a healthy and long life which runs as follows:

dānaśīladayāsatya

brahmacarya kṛtajñatāḥ /

rasāyanāni maitrī ca

puṇyamāyurvṛddhikṛdguṇāḥ // [137]

Generosity, kindness, truthfulness, celibacy, gratitude, elixirs, friendship, and merits are the factors which increase the duration of life. These are the factors which govern long life.

The third chapter named *asthivibhāgādhyāya* consists of 300 verses. This chapter describes the importance of bones in the human body thus:

ābhyantaragataissārairyathā tiṣṭhanti bhūruhaḥ

asthisāraistathā dehāḥ dhriyante dehinām dhruvam // [138]

Just as the trees survive with the help of sap inside like wise the humanbody substains with bone and marrow in it.

Classification of bones, Cartilages and their formation, etc. are explained in detail. The fourth chapter named *sandhivibhāgādhyāya* consists of 222 verses. In this chapter characteristics of joints of bones according to Āyurveda and modern view are dealt with in detail. According to Āyurveda the joints are of two types; movable and immovable:

asthnām tu sandhayo dvedha

sthirāsthiravibhedataḥ / [139]

The joints of bones are of two types – movable and immovable.

In the following verses modern view regarding the joints of bones is given:

bhavantyathā navīnānām mate bhūyo 'pi cāsthiraḥ /

īṣaccalāścalaśceti dvidhā tat trividhā iha /

sthirāḥ punastridhā bhinnāḥ saucaraucakakaikasāḥ // [140]

According to modern view movable joints are again divided into partially movable (Amphiarthrosis) and movable (Diarthrosis). These three main types of joints are mentioned here in the text. The immovable joints are again divided into sutura, (*saucaḥ*) gomphosis (*raucakaḥ*) and synchondrosis (*kaikasaḥ*).

The fifth chapter named *peśīvibhāgādhyāya* consists of 180 verses. In this chapter the muscular tissues and their functions and formalities are described in detail. Muscular tissue is defined as follows:

māmsam śarīragam sarvam mṛdulohitakesaraiḥ

nirmīyate māmsadharāmsarūpakalayāvṛtaiḥ //

prāyaḥ prasāritāste syuḥ sarve samkocanakṣamāḥ

sthitisthapakavantaśca svabhāvanmilitā mithaḥ // [141]

The muscular tissues in the human body are formed out of thin muscular fibres. The fibres are ordinarly of expanded, (*prasārita*) but are capable of contraction, (*saṅkocanakṣama*) and elasticity (*stihitisthāpakavantaḥ*) combined in various propositions.

The sixth chapter named *nāḷivibhāgādhyāya* consists of 308 verses. In this chapter classification of blood vessels, with their functions and structures is explained in detail. The classification of blood vessels is described thus:

dhamanyaśca sirā raktāyanyaśceti tridhā matāḥ

raktanālyo 'tra dhamaniḥ sthūlabhittistrikañcukaḥ // [142]

Blood vessels (*raktanālyaḥ*) are classified into three; arteries, (*dhamanyaḥ*) Veins (*sirāḥ*) and capillaries (*raktāyanyaḥ*). Arteries possess a threefold covering around them.

The seventh chapter named *aṅgakarmavibhāgādhyāya* consists of 268 verses. It deals with different cavities in the human body. This chapter begins with the classification of cavities as follows:

dve antarāle dehe 'smin paścimam ca purasthānam

karoti pṛṣṭhavamśāntargatam paścimamucyate // [143]

The human body consists of two large cavities (*antarāle*) named cerebrospinal (*paścimam*) cavity and Cranial Cavity (*purasthānam*).

After that all other cavities like oral cavity, thoracic cavity, etc; secretions like gastric juice, pancreatic juice, bile, etc; are mentioned.

The eighth chapter named *tantranāḍivibhāgādhyāya* consists of 426 verses. It deals with the functions of the nervous system in human body. The classification of nervous system under two sub division is given here for illustration:

tantaranāḍī, tantrayantram tantrapaddhatirityapi

ekārthakāni nāmāni tatra dve upapaddhati //

syātām, śirovamśīyādyā syātsvayamśāsinī parā // [144]

Nervous system (*tantra nāḍī*), which is otherwise known as *tantra yantra* or *tantra paddhati* is classified under two heads as cerebrospinal (*śirovamśīya*) and autonomic (*svayamśāsinī*).

The work ends with the personal details of the author:

vikhyāto 'jani rāmapārśvajavaro mṛdvāpikūlālaye

sakhyetasya varāhacaityasadane śrīpārvatīcābhavat /

dampatyoranayossutassamatanocchārīramārṣamguroḥ

samprītyā jagatāmanena bhavatātsaukhyardhimārgodayaḥ // [145]

Sri. Rāma Vārrier was well known in the Māṅkulaṅṅara family. Panninpalli Śrīpārvatī was his wife. The son of that couple (namely P.S Varrier) composed this *Aṣṭāṅgaśārīra* by the blessings of those elders. Let this opened the path of increasing the happiness of the world.

There is also a glossary given at the end of the text in the alphabetical order, which helps the students to acquaint with the modern terms and their Sanskrit equivalents easily.

Gūḍhārthabodhinī Commentary

It is a commentary on *Aṣṭāṅgaśārīra* by the author himself. The meanings of the verses that are explained in simple lucid Sanskrit intermingled with Modern English terms. It would help the traditional Āyurvedic scholars also to acquaint with modern medical terms and their methodology. An example from *Aṣṭāṅgaśārīra* is quoted here to illustrate the nature the commentary.

> *śirogrīvam madhyakāyo dvau*
>
> *bāhū dve ca sakthinī /*
>
> *ṣaḍaṅgamevamaṅgam*
>
> *tatpratyaṅganayanādikam //* [146]

śirogrīvam śiraśca grīvā ca śirogrīvamūrdhvāṅgāparaparyāyam / śirasaḥ prādhānyena dvāvamśau bhavataḥ mūrdhā mukham ca / tatra svabhāvataḥ saromā paścimā uttaraśca bhāgo mūrdhetyucyate / purobhāgo niromā (anāgatasmaśruṇām) mukham ca bhavati / madhyakāyo'ntarādhiḥ, tasyordhvakhaṇḍaḥ uttarādhiḥ adharakhaṇḍo adharādhiriti cābhidhīyate / dvau bāhū dve uttara śākhe (upper extremities) dve sakthinī, dve adharvaśākhe (lower extremities) evam aṅgam śarīram ṣaḍaṅgam prādhānyenāvayavaṣatkopalakṣitam / tatpratyaṅgam tasya śarīrasya pratyaṅgam avayavasyāvayavaḥ / nayanādikam / ādi śabdena hṛdayādiparigrahaḥ //

Thus it can be seen that this commentary is very useful for Āyurvedic scholars to acquaint them with the modern scientific findings of English medicine in a simple manner.

J. *Bṛhacchārīra*

Bṛhacchārīra is an extension of the work *Aṣṭāṅgaśārīra*, giving more emphasis to Anatomy and rectifying the mistakes crept in the original Āyurvedic texts in course of time. In the preface to the text P. S. Varrier observes thus:

na kevalamādhunikapāśātya śārīraśāstradviṣayānuddhṛtya prācīnabhāra tīyaśārīraśāstrasya nyūnatāpariharaṇārthamasya granthasya nirmāṇārambhaḥ, api tu, yāni śarīratatvānyāyurvede sādhāraṇairajñātānyanyathā vyākhyātāni ca santi teṣām sphuṭīkaraṇe pramādaparihāreṇa cāyurvedasya yāvacchakti pūrṇatāpādanāya taddvārā nikhilalokopakāritvakaraṇāya ca/ āyurvedavaidyānāmiva anyavaidyapraviṇānāmapyayamupakariṣyatīti cāsti me manorathaḥ / [147]*

The composition of this work is intended not only for the removal of the *lacunae* in the ancient Indian anatomy (*śārīraśāstra*) by drawing the material from the modern anatomical texts of the Westerners but also for the elucidation of these principles of anatomy in Āyurveda which are not known to ordinary people and which are interpreted in a different way and give a state of completeness to the Āyurveda by rectifying the inconsistencies to the best of my abilities. I hope that this will be of use not only to the practitioners of Āyurveda but also to the practitioners of other traditions of medicine.

Bṛhacchārīra is the first ever work written in Sanskrit, where systematic arrangement of human anatomy can be seen. It is not a mere translation of any modern work on embryology but a well planned adaptation of modern teachings. L. A. Ravivarma who wrote foreword to the text observes thus:

The author has taken pains to ensure that the imported teachings mingle freely and well with the ancient teachings so as to make a harmonious whole, where in, the new incorporations will appear more as amplifications and elaboration's on the older teachings than a new and alien importation. The following passage will serve to explain what I mean: *tarhi kināma śarīram I śīryate pratikṣaṇamapacīyate iti śarīram I upacayopāya sampattāvapi nirantarāpacīyamanatvam śarīratvamityarthaḥ I thatā dagddhyupacīyate pratikṣaṇamāhārādinetyasya dehatvamapyasti I evam ca upacīyamānatvasamānakālīnāpacīyamānatvam śarīrasāmānyalakṣaṇamiti phalito'rthaḥ I yujyate caitat I yatassarve jīvacchrīrāṃśaḥ sarvadāpi dhātvagnipākavaśāt svasvocitamannasārāṃśam gṛhītvopacayam jīrṇāṃśam parityajyāpacayam ca prayāntīti suviditam sūkṣmasadṛśam I etādṛśopacayāpacayajanakodhātvagnipāka eva saṅghaṭakavighaṭakātmakajīvyanupāka-* (constructive and destructive metabolism) *tveva varṇyate navīnaiḥ,*

Then what is it that is called *śarīra* (body). It is *śarīra* because it is exhausted every second (*śīryate apacīyate*). It means that the characteristic of *śarīra* is its waning away continuously even though there is the possibility of the means of growth. It is also *deha* in the sense that it grows with food etc; every movements. The resultant general definition of *śarīra* amounts that which has simultaneous waxing and waning. This definition holds good because it is known to persons of subtle insight that all the parts of the living body attain growth by extracting the essences of food according to their requirements, due to the nourishing elements and digestion through gastric fire, and undergo waning at the same time by discharging the digested elements. This combination of the nourishing elements and digestion through heat is described in terms of constructive and destructive metabolism by the modern thinkers).

How well the modern ideas of Anabolism, Catabolism and Metabolism have been incorporated can be seen from this passage.[148]

The text is written in simple Sanskrit verses so as to enable the aspirant to memorise them very easily. Another feature of the work is the illustration given in the text. The last but not least is the coining of new technical terms.

Bṛhacchārīra was published in two volumes. The first volume *Sṛṣṭiskandha* was published in 1942. It deals with embryology in 21 chapters. The second volume **Astiskandha** was published by S. R. Iyer in 1969. It consists of ten chapters.

Sṛṣṭiskandha

Sṛṣṭiskandha opens with the benedictory verse as follows.

> *dhanvantarim sudhāpāṇīm –*
>
> *anvaham praṇato 'smyaham /*
>
> *nanvantarārdro hyādhivyā-*
>
> *dhyanvayam vidhunoti yaḥ //* [149]

I daily bow to Lord Dhanvantari who carries ambrosia in hands who out of compassion removes all diseases and gives pleasure to us remove all diseases and giving in pleasure.

The first chapter deals with the division of subjects going to be described in the text. There the author states that the treatise is prepared after studying the old and new texts on treatment and proven by experience. Varrier further states that he wrote the work as for acquiring ultimate goal in life (*puruṣārtha*) sound health is necessary.

> *nānātantrāṇi samvīkṣya prācīnāni navāni ca*
>
> *sarveṣām puruṣārthānām śarīram sādhanam yataḥ*
>
> *tatastatparirakṣārtham śraddha kāryā 'khilairapi //* [150]

Since, the body is the means for all to attain the fourfold values of life every body should take interest in protecting it by consulting the texts on medicine, both old and new.

P.S Varrier further states that

cikitsāśāstramakhilam dehamuddiśya nirmitam

tasmāddehasya vijñāne vaidyasiddhiḥ pratiṣṭhitā // [151]

The whole lot of the science of therapy is formulated for the sake of this human body. Hence the success of a physicians depends upon the knowledge of human body.

In the second chapter named *aṅgavibhāga* different portions of the human body are describe thus:

śirogrīvam madhyakāyo

dvau bāhū dve ca sakthinī /

etānyaṅgāni dehasya

mukhyānyāhurmaharṣayaḥ // [152]

The portions of the body are divided into six. They are the head portion, consists of head and neck, the middle portion, two upper extremities two lower extremities.

It is interesting to note that the author quotes the same verse from the same named chapter in *Aṣṭāṅgaśārīra.*[153] In *Aṣṭāṅgaśārīra* he just mentioned the principles and concepts according to allopathy in Sanskrit verses but a detailed account of the above in prose and verse are given in *Bṛhacchārīra* with their English equivalents.

Eight main systems of the human body are described thus:

annanāḍī rasanāḍī raktanāḍī ca mūlataḥ

śvāsanāḍī mūtranāḍī śukḷanāḍyapyatha striyāḥ

rajonāḍī ca vartante tantranāḍī tu paścime // [154]

The systems of the human body are (1) *annanāḍī* (Alimentary system) (2) *rasanāḍī* (Lymphatic system) (3) *raktanāḍī* (Blood circulatory system) (4) *śvāsanāḍī* (Respiratory system) (5) *mūtranāḍī* (urinary system) (6) *śukḷanāḍī* (Male genital organs) (7) *rajonāḍī* (Female genital organs) and (8) *tantranāḍī* (Nervous system).

In addition to the above mentioned topics the chapter also contains detailed account of the organs like heart, brain, oval cavity, intestine, kidney etc. This chapter concludes with the verse thus:

yenaivamaṅgapratyaṅga

vibhāgo jñāyate dṛḍham /

ādyam śarīra śāstrasya

sopānam so 'dhigacchati // [155]

When one who acquires thorough knowledge about organs mentioned in the text, one enters in the branch of Anatomy.

The third chapter is nasmed as *bhūtavibhāgādhyāya*. This chapter begins with the description of five principal elements (*pañcabhūtas*) of body and explains how they take part in the formation of human body.

mahābhūtāni kham vāyu-

ragnirāpaḥ kṣitistathā // [156]

The *pañcabhūtas* (principal elements) of the body are *kham* (sky), *vāyu* (air), *agni* (fire), *āpaḥ* (water) and *kṣiti* (earth).

This chapter concludes with the verse giving emphasis to the need for the understanding of *pañcabhūta* as responsible for the formation of the human body.

śarīratatvavijñāne pañcabhūtavivecanam /

mukhyam bhavati yattasmin śiṣṭam jñānam pratiṣṭhitam // [157]

The knowledge of the *pañcabhūta* theory is necessary for proper understanding of human body; because the rest of the science is based on that.

The fourth chapter is called as *mūladravyavibhāgādhyāya*. In this chapter modern concept about the composition of human body is given as follows:

ākāśajaścārdrajaśca naitrajaḥ kārbaṇastathā /

gandhako bhāsvaraścaiva klorakāśaśca saptamaḥ //

mūladravyāṇyayalauhāni dehe saptaivamādiśet /

dṛśyante tānyamukhyatvāt gaṇitānyatra na pṛthak // [158]

ākāśaja (oxigen), *ārdraja* (hydrogen), *naitraja* (nitrogen), *kārbaṇa* (carbon), *gandhaka* (sulpher), *bhāsvara* (phospherous), *klorakāsa* (chlorine) are the seven principle constituent non-metallic elements responsible for the formation of human body.

Varrier points out that the constituent elements for the formation of body according to modern science and the *pañcabhūta* theory are complementary to each other:

173

evam navīnamate mūladravyāṇām tatsamyuktānāñcānekadhā vibhāge'pi teṣām sarveṣāmapi prācīnoktapañcamahābhūte (mahābhūtannāma pañcīkṛtam khādibhūtam) ṣvevantarbhāvo dṛśyate / na hi tadbhinnam kimapi navīnam dravyamupalabhyate / parantu teṣāmevāmśakakalpanayā pṛthaksvarūpakarmādīnām sūkṣmataram jñānam taissampāditamiti vastuto nānyonyavirodhaḥ / [159]

Thus although according to the modern view there is an analysis of the constituent elements to into their many forms, yet all of them can be included in the ancient theory of the five elements, i.e, the five elements as constituting the *pañcīkaraṇa* processes. There is nothing new other than that can be found. But the modern thinkers have discovered subtler and subtler facts about the nature of those elements by analysing their different aspects. In fact there is no mutual opposition between them.

This chapter concludes with the verse thus:

rasāyanam śarīrasya vibhāgam vetti yo bhiṣak /

sa cikitsāvidhau naiva muhyati vyādhisamśayāt // [160]

The physician (*bhiṣak*) who knows the chemistry of human body will not have any doubt at all during treatments.

The fifth chapter is named as *dhātuvibhāgādhyaya*. In this chapter sevan types of *dhātus* are described.

rasaraktamāmsamedomajjāno mastuluṅga śukle ca /

mukhyā dhātava ete mūlānyanyasya dhātuvargasya // [161]

rasa, rakta, māmsa, medas, majjā, mastuṅgam (nerve matter), *śukra* are the seven principal *dhātus* (constituents)

Different characteristics of *saptadhātus* are described in the remaining portions. This chapter concludes in the importance of this study of the *dhātuvibhāgādhyāya* thus:

dhātuvibhāgam samyak proktam jānāti yo 'gadaṅgāraḥ /

yadi so 'khilavaidyavarān jñānādativartate na citram tat // [162]

One who acquires thorough mastery over *dhātuvibhāga* portion mentioned here, will surpass all other physicians.

The sixth chapter is named as *pratīkavibhāgādhyāya*. It contains detailed description of different constituent elements and their characteristics, the proportions of different *dhatus* for the formation of human body are described thus:

> *dhātvādisaṅkarodbhūtā ye ye bhāgāśśarīragaḥ /*
>
> *pratyekato 'tra vijñeyaḥ pratīkāmstān pracakṣate //* [163]

The *pratīkas* are those which contained the knowledge about the various proportion of the human organs that are evolved by the combination of the elements.

This chapter concludes with the verse saying that one who studied *pratīkādhyāya* is able to do surgery.

> *pratīkān yo vijānāti pratyekam bāhyacakṣuṣā /*
>
> *sa eva śastrakarmāṇi kartum śaknoti netaraḥ //* [164]

One who understands the matter given in *pratīkādhyāya* through his eyes, alone is able to do surgery.

The seventh chapter is named as *dhātuparamāṇuvijñānīyādhyāyaḥ*. The characteristics of minute particles like *lohitasattva* (RBC), *yauvata* (ovum), garbhaka (corpuscles), etc. are described in detail. The text declares thus:

> *yo dhātuparamāṇūnām svabhāvam paṭhati svayam*
>
> *sa eva śaktastajjanyān dhātūn jñātum vibhāgataḥ //* [165]

One who acquires the knowledge of minute elements of the body, alone understands the composition of *dhātus*.

The eighth chapter is named as *rasādivijñānīyādhyāya*. In this chapter different particles of blood, lymphatic circulation (*rasaparivartanam*), lymph plasma (*rasaplāvika*), fibrinogen (*paiṛṇajanaka*) etc are described in detail.

The ninth chapter is named as *māmsadhātuvijñānīyādhyāya*. It deals with different types of muscular fibres and their functions.

The tenth chapter is named as *mastuluṅgadhātuvijñānīyādhyāya*. It deals with nervous system (*tantrayantra*), *madhyatantra* (central nervous system) etc in detail.

The eleventh chapter is named *tanudhātuvijñānīyādhyāya*. It deals with different type of skins, the covering of thyroid gland (*kākalagoḷa*) etc.

The twelfth chapter is named as *samyojakadhātuvijñānīyādhyāya*. It deals with different type of tissues in detail.

The thirteenth chapter is named as *asthidhātuvijñānīyādhyāya*. It deals with different categories of bones and their constituent elements in detail. The author concludes this chapter by giving emphasis to the need for the study of this portion.

>*asthisambandhino rogāḥ bahavassanti dāruṇāḥ /*
>
>*na te 'sthitatvavijñānādṛte sādhyaścikitsitum //*
>
>*tasmādasthnām samutpattirghaṭanāpoṣaṇakramāḥ /*
>
>*kendropakendrayogādyaścādau jñeyā bhiṣagvaraiḥ //* [166]

There are so many dangerous diseases connected with bones. The treatment is possible only when one knows the structure and characteristics of various bones thoroughly.

This section constitutes the entire second part of the text.

The fourteenth chapter is named as *garbhāvakrāntīya*. The ideal time for marriage is given here.

>*pūrṇaṣoḍaśavarṣāyām pañcavimśatikapumān*
>
>*putrārtham prayatataiṣa kālassatputrasiddhidaḥ //* [167]

Only a man who has completed 25 years and a woman who has attained the age of 16 years should only try for begetting a child. That is the right time for obtaining a healthy son.

The structures of spermatozoon (*pauruṣaḥ*), ovum (*yauvataḥ)* etc are given in detail. The origin of pregnancy, the structures of ectoderm (*bahirdharma*), endoderm (*antardharma*), etc. are also mentioned.

The fifteenth chapter is named as *garbhavṛddhikramavivaraṇādhyāya*. As the name indicates it deals with the development of the fetus in the initial stages of pregnancy. After discussing various views of Caraka, Suśruta and Vāgbhaṭa modern view about the development of fetus is described in detail. This chapter concludes with the diagram of the fetus in the second month.

The sixteenth chapter is named as *dehaiḍukapariṇāmavivaraṇādhyāya*. The development of various body cavities, the formation of vertebral column, and other developments occur up to the end of three months of pregnancy. These details are given with their diagrams.

The seventeenth chapter is named as *tantranā ḍīdhīndriya pariṇāmavivaraṇādhyāya*. The development of the *gordanāla* (Medulla spinals), the diagrams of the fetus at the fourth month, the formation of brain tube, eyes, etc. are explained in detail. This chapter concludes with the detailed description with diagram of the development of ears of the fetus at the end of the third month.

The eighteenth chapter is named as *nāḷīpaddhatipariṇāmavivaraṇādhyāya.* In this chapter formation and structure of blood vessels, erythrocytes, lymphocytes, heart tubes, heart etc are mentioned in detail.

The nineteenth chapter is named as *annanāḍiśvāsanāḍyoḥ pariṇāmavivaranādhyāyaḥ.* The formation of mouth, tongue, thyroid glands, platen tonsils, thymus, pituitary glands, craniopharyngeal canal, pharynx, rectum, anal canal, pancreas, respiratory organs, epiglottis, glottis, thyroid cartilage etc are described in detail.

The twentieth chapter is named as *dehaguhāmūtraśukḷarajonāḍīnām pariṇāmavivaraṇādhyāyaḥ.* The formation of *vastyupasthīyāṅgāni* (uro genital organs) viz. excretory organs (*visarjanārthāni*) and reproductive organs (*punarutpādanārthani*) are descried in detail. The formation of genital glands, fetes, epoophoron (*uporvara*), ductusaberrans (*upaśukḷavaha*), urogenital sinus, genital chord (*upasthasūtram*), vasdefferance (*śukḷapraṇāḷī*) are described. The separate diagrams of the female fetus and male fetus in the womb are given in detail.

The last chapter which is the 21st chapter is named as *garbhapurtivivaraṇā dhyāya.* In this chapter the development and changes in the fetus from first month to the ninth month are abridged in beautiful Sanskrit verses. In this chapter the movement of the child during the various stages of pregnancy is also mentioned. This text ends with paying homage to his preceptors thus:

> *vaidyagresaravāsudevadharaṇīdevasya sākṣādguroḥ*
>
> *vāryasyācyutanāmna āṅgalabhiṣagvargeśiturdhīmataḥ /*
>
> *vargīśasya ca satkṛpāphalamayaḥ skandho 'yamādyo bṛha-*
>
> *cchārīrasya mayā kṛtaḥ kṣitibhuvām bhūyātparam śreyase //* [168]

I have composed the first part of *Bṛhacchārīra* of the all human beings. This is the result of blessings from my teacher Acyuta Varrier who was the direct guru of Vāsudeva, the foremost among the physicans and my teacher Dr. Varghese who was well versed in modern medicine.

Asthiskandha

This second portion of *Bṛhacchārīra* consists of ten chapters exclusively dealing with only bones with the objective to give a specialised knowledge in that area. This has been stated at the beginning of the texts.

asthnām sūkṣmam sṛṣṭyādi svarūpam sṛṣṭiskandhe varṇitam /

idānīm viṣeṣavijñānārtham pratyekato asthivivaraṇamārabhyate // [169]

The origin of bones and their characteristics are already mentioned in *sṛṣṭiskandha*. For a specialised knowledge in this area (study of bones) an attempt is made here separately.

The first chapter is named as *pṛṣṭhavaṁśavivaraṇādhyāya*. Total number of bones in a human body according to Āyurveda and modern science is given here. The division of skeleton into two according to modern science is described here in detail thus: *dehasthasyaasthipañcarasyātra kaṅgāla iti samjñā / sa dvividhaḥ akṣakaṅkālaḥ upakaṅkālaśceti / tayorakṣakaṅkāle madhyakāyasyordhvāṅgasya ca sarvāṇyasthinyantarbhavanti / upakaṅkāle tu śākhānāmiti bhedaḥ //* [170]

The skeleton of the human body is named as *kaṅkāla* in Sanskrit. It is divided into two. *akṣakaṅkāla* (axial skeleton) and *upakaṅkāla* (Appendix skeleton).

The former consists of all bones in the thorasic region and latter consists of all other bones in the lower region. Classification of bones according to their shapes and the structure of the bones at the joints etc are mentioned here in this chapter in detail.

The second chapter is named as *śiraḥkapālavivaraṇa*. The structure of the skull (*śiro 'sthipañjaraḥ*) and its divisions into two as cranium (*karoṭi*) and face (*mukha*) and their structures are described with their diagrams in detail.

The third chapter is named as *itarakaroṭyasthivivaraṇa*. The remaining bones like temporal bones (*saṅkakāsthi*), etc. for the formation of human skull with their diagrams are described here in detail.

The fourth chapter is named as *mukhamaṇḍalāsthivivaraṇa*. It contains detailed description of the structures of the bone in the facial region (*mukhamaṇḍala*). Facial region is defined as the front portion of head except forehead:

lalāṭavarjitasya śirapurobhāgasya mukhamaṇḍalamiti samjñā // [171]

pṛṣṭavamśasya uttarārdhamavalambya tiṣṭhati śirosthipañjaraḥ /

sa karoti mukhamiti dvidhā vibhaktaḥ //

The fifth chapter is named as *samastaśirakaṅkālavivaraṇa*. In this chapter the external portion of the skull like corunal suture (*kairīta*) sagittal (*madhyamassāyaka*), lambdoidal (*paścimasīmanta*), etc., lower regions that is hard palate structure of nasal cavities (*nāsāguha*) etc. are described with diagrams in detail. The changes occurring in the skeleton in various stages of growth are also given here in detail.

The sixth chapter is named as *uro'sthipārśukavivaraṇa*. The classification and structure of sternum (*urosthi*), ribs (*pārśuka*), etc. are mentioned here in detail.

The seventh chapter is named as *amsacakravivaraṇādhyāya*. The bones coming under the Appendix skeleton (*upakaṅkala*) like acromion (*amsakūṭaḥ*), clavicles (*akṣake*), etc. are mentioned with diagram in detail.

The eighth chapter is named as *uttaraśākhāsthivivaraṇa*. It deals with the bones like humerus (*pragaṇḍāsthi*) the ones in the neck etc with structures in detail.

The ninth chapter is named as *kaṭīcakravivaraṇa*. It consists of the structure of hip joints and details of the bones for the formation of the hip portion. This chapter concludes with the structure and description of the pelvic girdle (*kaṭīcakra*) of male and female separately.

The tenth chapter is named as *adhaśśākhāsthivivaraṇa*. It contains the detailed description of femur (*pīvarāsthi*), the bones in the knee, the skeleton of the feet, the minute bones (*cartilages*) etc. in detail. The text concludes with the description of small bones in the human body especially bones in the ears. (*cartilage*).

A glossary is also given as an appendix to the text in the alphabetical order in Sanskrit. It will be helpful to the students to get English equivalents of Sanskrit words used in the text.

Other Works

The codification and dissemination of existing knowledge was an area to which P.S Varrier devoted considerable attention. For that purpose he wrote works like *Cikitsāsaṅgraha, Viṣūcikā, Dhanvantari* (Fortnghtly), and *Āryavaidyacaritram* in Malayalam.

Cikitsāsaṅgraha

It is a catalogue of medicines giving details about the usage, dosage and other necessary information. It enables even common man to consume them with out medical prescription.

Viṣūcikā

It is a work on cholera meant to popularise the ideas of Āyurveda regarding the disease of that time with its causes and cures. Once the area of Koṭṭakkal was got afflicted by that disease. Then Varrier saved many of the people by using Āyurvedic medicines.[172]

Āryavaidyacaritram

It was the first history of Āyurveda written in an Indian language. P.S Varrier and his cousin P.V Krishna Varrier combindly wrote it. It helps the common folk to know about the tenets of Āyurveda.

Dhanvantari

It was a fortnightly journal published by P.S Varrier from Koṭṭakkal on 1902. It served as a tongue of revitalization movement of Āyurveda in Kerala.[173] This provided an open forum for debates and discussions, as evident from some articles published in it.

K. VAIDYAMANORAMĀ

Vaidyamanoramā is an independent work on Āyurveda by a Keralite scholar. Details about the date and name of the author are not known. From the last *śloka* of the text it can be inferred that he is a devotee of Śiva.

adhunā śivapādasevakena

pṛthageṣā sakalāgamārtharūpā /

racitā bhiṣajām manoramā

januṣā rogasamāptaye samāptā // [174]

I, who am a devotee of Śiva, have dealt with separately the Āyurveda according to the authentic texts, in this work which is appealing to the physician, for the eradication of diseases of the beings.

Vaṭakkumkūr points outs that verses from *Vaidyamanoramā* are quoted by the author of *Sarvarogacikitsāratna*.[175] This shows the importance of the text. The text is divided into twenty two chapters named *adhikāra's. cikitsādhikāra, jvara, raktapitta, kāsa, arocakam, arśas, atisāram, mūtrakṛccham, vidradhi, mahodaram, kāmila, śopham, kuṣṭham, vātam, garbhiṇīcikitsā, bālacikitsā, netrarogacikitsā, karṇarogacikitsā, arbudam, guhyarogam, viṣacikitsā, rasāyana,* and *vājīkaraṇa* treatments are dealt in detail. But the emphasis is given to the *cikitsādhikāra*. The author claimes that the medicines prescribed in the text are prepared out of ingredients, which are cheap and easily available.

sulabhā subhagabheṣajāni siddhā

nyamṛtasamānaphalāni yāni yāni /

sakalagadaharāṇi mānavāna-

miha kathitāni bhavanti tāni tāni //[176]

The medicines that are very effective and prepared out of easily available and cheap materials are mentioned here.

The description of *masūri* (small pox) disease in the 11th *paṭala* is interesting.

śīghrameṣa prabhāveṇa saṅkrāmati nārannaram /

bhayabaibhatsya śokādyāssaṅkrame hetavaḥ smṛtāḥ //

āturāṅgasamudbūtam viṣabījam marutvatā /

Vyāpāritam tatsahasā vyāpnoti jagatītale //

Varjayedrogasānnidhyam samparkam paricārakaiḥ /

taducchiṣṭāśanam yatnāt tat kathāsmaraṇam thatā // [177]

Because of fear, grief, etc., small pox spreads easily from one man to another. Again the disease spreads when exposed to the wind (which carry *viṣabījam* or Virus coming from the patient. So their contact should be avoided even by their assistants, their presence or remembrance of their deeds, should be avoided and it is prohibited to take meals taken by them at all costs.

Thus it can be concluded that the physicians should have the clear understanding of the diseases and do their treatment out of careful observation at that time.

L. *KAUTUKACINTĀMAṆI*

It is a work by a Keralite, which can be concluded from the internal evidences from the text.[178] It contains 160 chapters. All chapters are technically known as *paṭalas*. At the end of the 10th *paṭala* there is a colophon thus;

> *iti siddhanāgārjunaviracite kautukacintāmaṇau daśamaḥ paṭalaḥ.*[179]

This is the tenth chapter of *Kautukacintāmaṇi* by Siddhanāgārjuna.

From this the author's name can be inferred as *Siddhanāgārjuna*. Vaṭakkumkūr opines that from the name *Siddhanāgārjuna* one can infer that the author is a Buddhist.[180]

The text contains different kinds of *mantras,* medicines, oral medicines, etc., in detail. It also contains the preparation of medicines out of the herbs that are available only in Kerala. It contains verses in Malayalam also. An example is given here for illustration.

> *mārjārasya malam tālum*
>
> *piṣṭvā mūṣika māli pol. //* [181]

Vaṭakkumkūr points out that *tālu* is the famous tālu tree in Kerala. It is also interesting to note that in this work, *Vṛkṣāyurveda* is dealt in detail.

References

BHEṢAJAPADDHATI is a published work yet it is not noticed in any of the published works dealing with the history of Āyurveda either in English or Malayalam.

1. Puruṣottaman Nambūtiri, *Bheṣajapaddhati* I-2.

2. *Ibid.*, I –1.

3. *Ibid.*, I – 2.

4. *Ibid.*, IV – 102.

5. *Ibid.*, Introduction -II.

6. *Ibid.*, I - 4 – 8.

7. *Ibid.*, I – 9 –16.

8. *Ibid.*, I – 17 –31.

9. *Ibid.*, I – 32 – 44.

10. *Ibid.*, I –1-44-59.

11. *Ibid.*, II – 1 – 14.

12. *Ibid.*, II – 15-16.

13. *Ibid.*, II – 17-27.

14. *Ibid.*, II – 28-30.

15. *Ibid.*, III – 31-38.

16. *Ibid.*, III – 2-3.

17. *Ibid.*, Introduction –III.

18. *Ibid.*, IV 1- 16.

19. *Ibid.*, IV – 17-20.

20. *Ibid.*, IV – 21 –27.

21. *Ibid.*, IV – 61-68.

22. *Ibid.*, IV – 73-80.

23. *Ibid.*, III –34, *Aṣṭāṅgahṛdaya*, sūtrasthāna, IV –1

    Ibid., III –30, *Aṣṭāṅgahṛdaya*, sūtrasthāna, XIV –5.

    Ibid., IV –29, *Aṣṭāṅgahṛdaya*, sūtrasthāna, XV –9,10.

    Ibid., IV –82, *Aṣṭāṅgahṛdaya*, cikitsāsthāna, XXI –55.

24. *Ibid.*, I-2.

25. *Aṣṭāṅgahṛdaya,* Sūtrasthāna, III –2.

26. *Bheṣajapaddhati,* II-33.

27. *Ibid.*, III-55A.

28. *Sahasrayoga,* p. 45.

29. *Bheṣajapaddhati,* III-72A.

30. *Sahasrayoga,* p. 58.

31. *Bheṣajapaddhati,* II-15.

32. *Ibid.*, II –24.

33. *Ibid.*, III –13.

34. *Ibid.*, III- 19.

35. *Ibid.*, III –51.

36. *Ibid.*, III –52.

37. *Ibid.*, III-72 A.

38. *Ibid.*, IV –90.

39. *Ibid.*, II –32.

40. *Ibid.*, IV –101.

41. Dr. Raghavan Thirumulppad *(ed), Rasavaiśeṣika,* Preface, p.ii.

42. N.V. Krishnankutty Varriar, *Āyurvedacaritram,* p. 346.

43. *iti bhadanatanāgārjunasya pravrājitasya vaidyendrasya rasavaiśeṣikasūtrasya narasimhakṛtam bhāṣyam samāptam I*

44. Dr.Raghavan Thirumulppad, *Rasavaiśeṣika,* Preface, p.ii.

45. *Ibid.*

46. *Ibid.*, sūtra 1/4.

47. *Ibid.*, sūtra 1/132.

48. *Ibid.*

49. *Ibid.*, 3/61.

50. *Aṣṭāṅgahṛdaya* – uttarasthāna, 40/81.

51. *Rasavaiśeṣika,* 4/70.

52. *Ibid.*, 4/71.

53. N.V Krishnankutty Vārrier, *Āyurvedacaritram,* p. 346.

54. Dr. Raghavan Thirumulppad, *Rasavaiśeṣika,* Preface, p.IV.

55. *Ibid.,* 1/31.

56. Aravattattazhikattu K.V Krisnan Vaidyan & Anakkalil S. Gopalapillai (editors) *Sahasrayoga;* Preface, 1.

57. *Ibid.,* p. 122.

58. *Ibid.,* p. 1.

59. *Ibid.,* p.103.

60. *Ibid.*

61. *Ibid.*

62. *Ibid.,* p.145.

63. *Ibid.,* p. 224.

64. *Ibid.,* p. 467.

65. *Ibid.,* p. 460.

66. M. Duraiswami Ayyangar (ed), *Tantrasārasaṅgraha* Preface- I.

67. *Ibid.*

68. *Ibid.,* p.iv.

69. *Tantrasārasaṅgraha,* I/2.

70. *Ibid.,* I/3.

71. Dr.N.V.P Unithiri (ed) *Tantrasārasaṅgraha,* p.461.

72. *Ibid.,* Introduction, p.VIII.

73. Raja K. Kunjunni, *CKSL,* p.263.

74. Sāmbaśivaśāstri (ed), *Hṛdayapriyaḥ* Preface, II.

75. Vaikkam Pāccumūttatu, *Sukhasādhaka* biography, p.16.

76. *Ibid.,* p.16.

77. *Hṛdayapriyaḥ,* preface, IV.

78. Vaikkam Pāccumūttatu, *Hṛdayapriya,* IV/12/57.

79. *Ibid.,* I/1/6.

80. *Ibid.,* I/16/29.

81. *Ibid.,* I/16/29.

82. Sāmbaśivaśātri (ed), *Hṛdayapriya*, Preface, III.

83. See FN, 78.

84. Abhinavagupta, *Abhinavabhāratī*.

85. Vāgbhaṭa, *Aṣṭāṅgahṛdaya*, I/2/1.

86. Vaikkam Pāccumūttatu. *Hṛdayapriya*, I/1/22.

87. *Ibid.*, I/2/54.

88. *Ibid.*, II/3/22.

89. *Ibid.*, IV/12/56.

90. Vaikkam Pāccumūttatu, *Sukhasādhaka*, XII/3/61.

91. *Ibid.*, I/1/1.

92. *Ibid.*, /XII/3/62.

93. Dr. Raghava Varrier & Rajan Gurukkal, *Keralacaritram,* p.15.

94. *Ibid.*, p. 25.

95. *KSC* Vol. IV, p. 301.

96. *Ibid.*

97. *Dhārākalpa*, Benedictory verse.

98. *Ibid.*, 1.

99. *Ibid.*, 2.

100. *Ibid.*, 3.

101. One *hasta* approximately equal to 45.72cm.

102. One *aṅgula* approximately equals to 1.95cm.

103. *Dhārākalpa* —6.

104. *Ibid.*, 14.

105. *Ibid.*, 34.

106. *Contribution of Kerala to Sanskrit Literature.* p. 258.

107. *Keralīya Samskṛta Sāhitya Caritram.* IV p. 579.

> *Yasyopanāma nijadāsapadam gatasya*
>
> *Vāgdāsa ityakṛt kaścana siddhayogī /*
>
> *rameti nāma ca yathāgamavedavidvā*
>
> *nānandanāthapādaśekharatamayāsīt //*

108. This text edited by Anekkalil Gopalapillai posses a slight change in the name as *Ārogyarakṣākalpadruma.*

109. *Ārogyakalpadruma* – I –1

110. *Ibid.,* p. 35.

111. *Ibid.,* III p.45.

112. *Ibid.,* V p. 83.

113. *Ibid.,* IX p.133.

114. *Ibid.,* IX p.137.

115. *Ibid.,* XI p.151.

116. *Ibid.,* XV p. 243.

117. *Ibid.,* XXVI p. 399.

> *pṛthagevākṣirogāṇām*
> *cikitsānyatra vakṣyate /*
> *savistaā thatāpyatra*
> *samkṣepāt sābhidhīyate //*

118. *Ibid.,* p. 404.

> *varāmadhukadārvībhirnnāli kerodake sṛte*
> *pādāvaśiṣṭe pūtetha pākena ghanatām gate /*
> *pādāmśatulyamadhvāḍhye madhupādāmśasammitam*
> *ślakṣṇīkṛtam rajaḥ pītarohiṇyāḥ paṭututhayoḥ /*
> *tulyam tatṣoḍaśāmśe tadanyatarasamyutam*
> *karpūrañca ladaṣṭāmśamitañca maricam rajaḥ /*
> *samyojya yojayedakṣṇordvaudvauvindu tataḥ prage*
> *sāyamcāśu prayogoyamakṣipākam niyacchati /*
> *jalasrāva kaphasrāvanaktāndhyatimirādikān*
> anyāmśca dāruṇān rogān kṣiprameva śamannayet. //

119. *Ibid.,* XXXX. 548.

> *atrabālārthamuddiṣṭā*
> *yogā yojyāśca yūnyapi /*
> *ityekenobhayam siddham*
> *gṛhyatām tena madvacaḥ //*

120. *Contribution of Kerala to Sanskrit Literature,* p.259.

121. P.S Varriar, *Bṛhacchārīra* I/1/1.

122. Thanu.V.G, 'Contribution of Vaidyaratnam P.S Vārrier', *Indian scientific tradition,* Edited by Dr.N.V.P Unithiri.

123. K.N Panicker, 'Indegenous Medicine and cultural Hegemony'. A study of the Revitalization movement in Kerala', *Samagra Souvenir,* 1996, p.66.

124. *Dhanvantari,* 16 August 1913.

125. *Ibid.,* Vol XII.

126. *Carakasamhitā, śarīrasthāna* 6.

127. See Appendix for details.

128. P.S Varriar, *Aṣṭāṅgaśārīra* I-1.

129. *Ibid .,* I-2.

130. *Ibid.,* I –9.

131. *Ibid.,* I – 12.

132. *Ibid .,* I –30, 31.

133. *Ibid.,* II-1.

134. *Ibid .,* II –82.

135. *Ibid .,* II –122.

136. *Ibid .,* II –125-6.

137. *Ibid.,* II –187.

138. *Ibid.,* III – 1.

139. *Ibid.,* IV-1.

140. *Ibid .,* IV –3.

141. *Ibid .,* V-1.

142. *Ibid .,* VI –1.

143. *Ibid .,* VII –1.

144. *Ibid .,* VIII –1.

145. *Ibid.,* I concluding verse, p. 472.

146. *Ibid.,* I *Gūḍhārthabodhinī* (commentary) p. 23.

147. P.S Varriar, *Bṛhacchārīra* I-1, Preface –vii.

148. *Ibid.*, I, forward by L. A. Ravivarma.

149. *Ibid.*, I I/p.1.

150. *Ibid.*

151. *Ibid.*

152. *Ibid* ., p.3.

153. *Aṣṭāṅgahṛdaya,* II –1.

154. *Bṛhacchārīra,* p. 6.

155. *Ibid* ., p.11.

156. *Ibid.*

157. *Ibid.,* p.14.

158. *Ibid.*

159. *Ibid.,* p.16.

160. *Ibid.*

161. *Ibid* ., p.18.

162. *Ibid.,* p.21.

163. *Ibid.*

164. *Ibid.,* p.32.

165. *Ibid.,* p.38.

166. *Ibid.,* p.74.

167. *Ibid.,* p.75.

168. *Ibid.,* p.190.

169. *Ibid.,* II p.1.

170. *Ibid.*

171. *Ibid.,* p.41.

172. Kizhedatt Vasudevan Nair, *Vaidyartnam P.S Varrier, A Biography,* pp. 39 –44.

173. Dr. K. N Panikkar, 'Indigenous Medicines and Cultural Hegemony', *Culture, Ideology and Hegmony,* p.162.

174. *Vaidyamanoramā,* p.315, *KSSC* Vol -I, p.513.

175. *KSSC,* Vol –3, p.522.

176. *Vaidyamanoramā*, p. 316, KSSC Vol-1, p.514.

177. Vaidyamanoramā, p. 286.

178. *KSSC,* Vol-1 p.514.

179. *KautukacintāmaṇI,* Colophon chapter X.

179. *KSSC,* Vol —1, 514.

180. *Ibid.*

Chapter 7

SANSKRIT SOURCES OF MALAYALAM TREATISES IN ĀYURVEDA

So far we have discussed Sanskrit works on Āyurveda popular in Kerala as well as written by Keralite authors. There are also a number of Malayalam works in Āyurveda. Most of the Malayalam works on Āyurveda directly or indirectly rely on Sanskrit *Samhitā* texts. But some of them represent the Kerala traditional Āyurveda before the coming of Sanskrit *Samhitās.* Text like *Sindūramañjarī* represents the siddha tradition. A general study of this works is also attempted in this chapter. As this is necessary to understand the impact of Sanskrit treatises on Keralas Āyurveda fully.

Cikitsāmañjarī

It is an independent work from Kerala in Maṇipravāla style, The text is also known as *Cikitsāṅgaprakāśinī.*

cikitsāmañjarī seyam cikitsāṅgaprakāśinī

anutsāryaprayogārhaiḥ samuddhārya mayocyate. [1]

Cikitsāmañjarī (also known as *Cikitsāṅgaprakāśinī*) is a collection of some most useful (medicines) by me (from authentic texts of Āyurveda.)

Vaṭakkamkūr in his *KSSC* points out that the author of this work is one Pulāmanthol Moos, without giving any reference.[2] But in the preface to the present text which is edited by D. Sreeraman Namboodiri and K.G Gopalapillai, it is said that the author and date of the work are not known. Vaṭakkamkūr also states that the work is incomplete and the text is only up to *mukharoga*

(Facial diseases).[3] But the present text contains the all topics in detail. In the preface to the text K.G Gopalapillai declares that the present text is based on two manuscripts got one from the son of Āranmula Nāṇattuvīttil Kochuraman Pillai named Krishna Pillai and another from the nephew of Āranmula Kochuraman Pillai named M.P Narayana Pillai.[4] So it is safer to say that Vaṭakkamkūr got a chance only to see that a portion of the text.

Cikitsāmañjarī is popular among the Kerala physicians as *Valiyamañjarī*. Even though it is an independent work, it heavily depends on *Aṣṭāṅgahṛdaya*, *Aṣṭāṅgasamgraha* and *Carakasamhitā*. The experience of the author in the treatment and some special preparations of Kerala are scattered here and there in the text. For eg. While prescribing the medicines for the ulcer in the abdomen of infants a special preparation is given thus:

> *Pūkkulāyāḥ rase siddham yaṣṭrī jīrakakalkkitam /*
>
> *Vidhinā neyy kuṭīccāl vayattil puṇṇaliccīṭum. // 5*

If one takes the medicine prepared with the juice of the Coconut flower with *Yaṣṭrī* (liquorice) *Jīrakam* (cumin), boiled ghee as ingredients, that cures ulcer in the stomach.

It also contains *snehasvedādicikitsā* which exists only in Kerala. It also contains some shortcut methods (*Kurumkauśalam*) of Keralities. An example is given to illustrate that from the end of the text. The medicine prescribed for healing the cracks in the feet is given thus:

> *cuṭṭeṇṇayil kuzhaccīṭṭu pulintoliyiṭām pade /*
>
> *āṭṭinte kāṣṭhavum kūṭṭām kālvillunnatozhiññupom //* [6]

The outer cyst of the tamarind fruit is roasted in fire and made into powder and then that powder is mixed with gingerly oil and the excretion of the goat. When that is applied to the feet, it will cure the cracks in the feet.

Thus the text is a mixture of the medicines from the authentic texts and those from the experiences of the author.

Sarvarogacikitsāratna

The text available now is with the *sujananandini* commentary by Anekkalilil. S.Gopalapillai published through Devi book stall, Kotungallor, (the sixth Edition on July 2002). This text is also popular among the Kerala physicians. It consists of an account of the causes of diseases and the treatments and of details about what are the curable diseases, what are incurable diseases etc. The text begins with a *śloka* on *pañcabhūtotpatti.* (origin of five primary elements) The origin of *pañcabhūtas* is described thus:

akṣarāt kham tato vāyu vayoragni tato jalam

udakāt pṛthvī jātā bhūtānāmeva sambhavaḥ. / [7]

The five principal elements are formed as follows:

From *akṣara* (constant; the Brahman) *kham* (sky) was produced, from this sky *Vāyu* (air), from air *agni* (fire), from fire *jalam* (water), and from water earth.

This is the idea of bhūtotpatti found in the Upaniṣads. For instance *Bṛhadāraṇyaka* says - ātmanaḥ ākāśaḥ sambhūtaḥ ākāśād vāyu, vāyoragni, angerāpaḥ, adbhyaḥ pṛthvī, pṛthvībhyo annam, annād retaḥ...[8]

The work describes the qualities of coconut thus:

nālikeram guru snigdham

vātaghnam svādu śītalam /

balamāmsapradam hṛdyam

bṛmhaṇam vastiśodhanam. // [9]

The coconut which is heavy and oily, destroys *vāta*, is tasty and cool, gives energy to body and heart, and felicitates purgation also.

It is interesting to note that there is only a slight change made by the author in the *śloka* in *Aṣṭāṅgahṛdaya.* [10] It also gives several synonyms to the medicines thus:

cikitsitam hitam pathyam

prāyaścittam bhṣagjitam /

bheṣajam śamanam śastam

paryāyaiḥ smṛtamauṣadham. // [11]

cikitsita, hita, pathya, prāyaścitta, bhiṣagjjita, bheṣaja, śamana, śasta etc are synonyms to medicine.

The above *śloka* is taken from *Aṣṭāṅgahṛdaya*[12] without giving any reference by author. Thus it can be said that this text is mainly based on *Aṣṭāṅgahṛdaya.*

Bālacikitsā — A

This work is published by Vidyārambham publishers, Mullakkal, Alleppy. The work available now is the 3rd edition of the text published in 1993 June. The details about the date and name of the author are not known. N.V Krishnankutty Varrier points out that it a collection of medicines used in the different houses (*Gṛhavaidya*) of Kerala.[13] He further clarifies that the oils like *kombañcādi*, *āsālyādi*, etc and the *kaṣāya* (decoction) used for the treatment of the mother after delivery, the *puliṅkuzhampu,* etc are mentioned in this work.[14]

The text consists of five parts. The first part is named as *garbhacikitsā* (the treatment of pregnancy), the second is named as *bālanidāna* (causes for the diseases in children and their treatment. The third part is named as *kuṭṭi pirannuvīṇiṭumnālmutal uṇṭākunna upadravam*. It consists of the treatment of child up to 16 years. The fourth part is named as *bālapīḍācikitsā*. It also consists of the description of different diseases and their treatment. The fifth chapter is named as *karappanucikitsā*. It deals with different types of skin diseases and their treatment. The text is very popular among Keraliya physicians. The text also contains recipes prescribed in *Aṣṭāṅgahṛdaya*.

Sarvarogacikitsānūl

The available text is the 5th Edition, published by John Alexander on January 1996 from Vidyarambham publishers, Alleppy. N.V Krishnankutty Varrier observes that the text consists of several special treatments of Kerala.[15] The text consists of two parts. In the first part the organs of the human body, their relations, and the diseases and treatments are described. In the second part named as *Vaidyanikṣepasaṅgraha* the ingredients (recipes) of the medicines described in the former chapter are described. The style of the work deserves special mention. To illustrate this a small portion from the beginning of the text is given here.

Toṇṇūttāraṅgulam tante viral koṇṭu śarīravum atinte madhyabhāgattu mūlādhāramayatu mūlādhārattiṅgalninnu suṣumnānāḍimelpāṭe kapālapadmattilolam cennu muṭṭiyirippatu... ... ...[16]

The height of a person is described as 96 times of length his finger. The *mūlādhāra* is situated in the centre of his body length. The *suṣumnā* (spinal chord) touches the Kapāla.

The author himself states that the text is prepared after collecting materials from *Aṣṭāṅgahṛdaya, Yogamañjarī, Mālikāmañjarī* and *Vaidyamanoramā, Yogāmṛta*, etc.

Mahāsāram

This book is edited by Dr. M.K Vaidyar, retired senior professor of Āyurveda College of Indigineous Medicine, Madras. This is available at Government Oriental Manuscripts Library, Madras. *Mahāsāram* is based on a single paper manuscript preserved in the Govt. Oriental Manuscript Library, Madras and described under D.No. 279. The book was published on 5-3-1951. In *Mahāsāram,* the author himself states that the *yogas* prescribed in this work are a collection of successful *yogas* available at that time.

> *Yādṛśam pustakam dṛṣṭam tādṛśam likhitam mayā /*
>
> *santaḥ samīkṣya gṛhnantu guṇam vā doṣameva vā //* [17]

The matter in this work is written according to the (authentic) texts on Āyurveda, let the scholars go through it carefully and find out the merits and demerits.

The subject matter of this work can be seen as classifiable under two heads, one dealing with *Vaidyaśāstra* (Medicine) and other with *Mantraśāstra (Bhūtavidyā).* In the first section on medicine which is studied in detail has the following chapters:

1) *Viṣacikitsā* dealing with various kinds of poisons

2) *Marmavibhāga and cikitsā* dealing with various kinds of important parts of human body and healing.

3) *Apasmāracikitsā* dealing with various kinds of *apasmāras.* In classical texts like *Aṣṭāṅgahṛdaya* only four types are explained. In this thirty-four types are explained. But individual symptoms are not given. The author has narrated many *yogas* with good result in the treatment.

4) *Bālacikitsā* dealing with paediatry, contains six *bhāgas* (chapters). First *bhāga* (chapter) contains the preparation of *Puliṅkuzhampu;* a special preparation of Keralite physicians.

5) Various prescriptions-prescriptions evolved out of his own experiences. The author has complied certain effective *yogas* (recipes) for different diseases. Some secret *yogas* (recipes) are also made available in this chapter. Some of them are (1) *Velīparuttiyāṭī virecana tailam* (2) *Āraṇya tulasī partādi tailam.*

6. *Balikarmams and Mantras* connected with *Bālacikitsa*. In this chapter *Mantras* and *Balikarmams (incantations and rituals)* starting from the birth up to 16th year are explained.

Vaidyasārasaṅgraha

This work is edited and published by T. Chandrasekharan, Curator, Government Oriental Manuscripts Library, Madras, in 1955. It consists of eight chapters. The manuscript has lacunae after the 7th chapter. All the miscellaneous topics found at the ends of the original manuscript have been included under Chapter VIII. This is a treatise on the treatment of the diseases of children. The first chapter deals with effective principles of pregnancy and treatments in each month. Some Mantras for painless delivery, also mentioned here. The second chapter deals with treatment of children for the Abdomen pain, *nābhiccheda*, etc. Other chapters explain various kinds of children and their diseases. The influence of *Aṣṭāṅgahṛdaya* can be seen while dealing with diseases of children.

Viṣavaidyasāravum viṣacikitsayum

The book is edited by Dr. A. Raman, Retired Vice-principal of S.A College Hospital at Culcutta. This book is also named as *Viṣavaidyampāṭṭu*. The work consists of two parts dealing with toxicology and the therapeutics with toxicosis respectively.

Both the parts deal at length about *dūtalakṣaṇas* ie., the ancient practice, by which the nature and outcome of the case is ascertained in advance by sending the messenger who brings the news of illness.

This also gives the *sādhyāsādhyalakṣaṇas* the determination of the curability or incurability of a disease by seeing the symptoms of the patient. Mention is also made about other insect bites. It appears that many prescriptions are adopted from the knowledge and practice prevalent amongst the old villagers of Kerala.

It is not possible to say as to who is the author. But in a manuscript made available from Tripunithura the author of *Viṣavaidyasārampāṭṭu* is mentioned as Koṭṭayattu Rājā.

Bālopacāra

It gives detailed explanation for the treatment of children. The book is mainly meant for mothers as it gives some basic principles of childcare. It was first edited in 1913 AD by Vellackal Narayana Menon, Bharatavilasam Printers, Trissur. The text contains eight chapters. In the first three chapters general diseases of the children up to six months and their remedies are described. The fourth chapter describes different types of *vraṇas* (injuries or wounds) in children and their treatments. The fifth chapter deals with the diseases pertaining to neck and the organs above the neck and their treatments. The sixth chapter explains the importance of breast feeding. The seventh chapter explains different types of *dhūpana* (disinfectants) *mantras,* etc. The eighth chapter deals with various types of diseases in adults and *yantras* to protect from diseases. The personal details about the author are unknown.

Garbhacikitsā

Dr. N. Madhava Menon has critically edited the work with introduction and notes on 1949 at Madras. Though the title is *Garbhacikitsā* it includes such things as menstrural periods, conception, pre-natal cure, treatment after childbirth, treatment of certain infantile diseases especially *karappan* (A type of skin disease).

There are six chapters in this book. The first chapter deals with mensus cycle, pregnancy, abortion, etc and their treatments. The second chapter deals with Paediatry. The third chapter deals with some special treatments for children. The fourth chapter includes diseases of children starting from birth up to 16 years. The fifth chapter is exclusively devoted to the disease called *karappan* ie., *visarpa* in Sanskrit. The sixth chapter deals with the treatment for constipation, urinary problems, jaundice, etc in detail. The date and personal details about the author are not known.

Cikitsakacintāmaṇi (Vaidyasaṅgraha)

The work was published on 1936 by K.G. Paramesvaran Pillai from Kollam. The author is 'Pandarathu Narayan Pillai Asan, Manamboor, Chirayankeezhu. Asan took birth in a traditional Āyurvedic family practicing *Viṣavaidya*. He is also called as *Paṇḍārattāsān*. The author gives an account of the special treatments out of his own experience. For eg. he advices the use the paste of *pāṣāṇa* for piles treatment.[18]

The work consists of two parts each with seven chapters containing about 500 *yogas* (recipes) in all. The first part contains details about diseases and in the second part treatment is prescribed. The author has collected 250 *yogas* (recipes) from the authentic texts and 250 from his personal experience. The date of the author is not known.

Agastyavaidyacandrikā

This text belongs to the Siddha tradition of Āyurveda. Kerala Āyurveda is a mixture of the medicinal elements in the authentic texts like *Aṣṭāṅgahṛdaya*, *Aṣṭāṅgasaṅgraha*, *Carakasamhitā* etc, and the medicines already available here before the reaching of the Sanskrit texts and Siddha tradition. This text conforms to the view that most of the medicines used in Kerala as *gṛhavaidyas* belonged to this Siddha tradition.

The Editor of the text is Vatayattukotta. K. Paramesvaran Pillai. The text available now is the fifth Edition published from Devi Bookstall Kotungallor on February 1998. In the introduction to the text the author declares that even though the text is named as *Agastyavaidyacandrikā*, it contains the medicinal preparations of other *siddhācāryas* and the effective medicines from his own experience also.[19]

The text contains 14 chapters in all. The first chapter contains detailed description of 'muppicunnam'. *Muppu* is the technical word to denote three type of salts. *muppu* is again divided into two *kalpamuppu* and *vaidyamuppu*. *Kalpamuppu is* a variety of salt used to strengthen our body; while 'vaidyamuppu' used for treatment of diseases. The latter is termed as 'muppucunnam' The descrimination and proper application of 'muppu' is said to be the secret of *vaidyakala* (treatment).

In the second chapter the preparation of *Agastyarkuzhampu*, the duties of a physician and the duties (deeds) of a patient are described. It is interesting to note here that there is an advice to the physicians that if the disease is unknown to him he should not treat that patient.[20] There is also an advice to the patient that if he is rich he should give proper fees to the physician. Otherwise he will fall into the hell. In the following chapters different types of *sindhūras, bhasmas* which are effective in the treatments are dealt with in detail.

Some medicines in *Keralīyagṛha's (gṛhacikitsā)* are mentioned in this text which shows the influence of Siddha tradition in Kerala Āyurveda. For eg., the preparation of hair oil for cold;. [21] Ingredients mentioned for this are the juice of *kaññuṇṇi (Trailing eclipta)* – half *iṭaṅgazhi* ginger oil, one *iṭaṅgazhi* the juice of *karinoccila* (five leaved chaste tree), – half 'itangazhi' when mixed with *satakuppa* (Dill), and boiled with powders of Cardomon and camphor will give an oil in black colour which will cure cold and head ache.

Mātaṅgalīlā

The text is composed by Thirumangalath Nilakanthan Musad on *Hastyāyurveda*. The text consists of twelve chapters. The chapters in the text are technically called as *paṭalas*. The text begins with the following verse:

> *mātaṅgavaktram praṇipatya dṛṣṭvā*
>
> *mātaṅgaśastram munipuṅgavoktam /*
>
> *mātaṅgalīlā caritāntarātmā*
>
> *mātaṅgalīlām racayāmi tāvat //.* [22]

The text is composed by me after seeing the *Mātaṅgaśāstram* of a sage. The text contains *nagotpatti* (origin of elephants) good and bad sign, different types of diseases etc in detail: Details about the author are not known.

Bālacikitsā- B

The text was written by Mandambeth Kunkatti Kunjiraman and published from Imperial Printers, Kannur, in 1923. The author explains that this is a collection of treatments available in *Ārogyakalpadruma, Aṣṭāṅgahṛdaya, Yogāmṛtam* etc., translated into Malayalam. Again he says that only effective treatments are taken into consideration. The author claims that the primary purpose of the book is to give a better understanding of diseases of the children to the parents.

Sindūramañjarī

The work is composed by Pazhznellippurath taikkatt Narayanan Musad of *aṣṭavaidya* clan in the later half of the 11th century ACE. Vaṭakkamkūr Raja Raja in his *K.S.S.C* mentioned this work with another name *Rasamañjarī*.[23] The present text is published by S.N.A publications, Trissur in the year 1994. The work belongs to *Siddha* tradition. Dr. Raghavan Thirumulppad in his introduction to *Sindūramañjarī* wonders how an Aṣṭavaidya can compose a work in the *Siddha* tradition. Dr. Raghavan Thirumulppad suggests that Narayanan Moos might have got the knowledge from some *Siddhas* who had visited the illam because *Aṣṭavaidyas* were popular as followers of *Aṣṭāṅgahṛdaya*. Raghavan Thirumulppad cited the following verse to substantiate this :

> *Keralīya janaṅṅalkkāṇṭariyān veṇṭi sādaram*
>
> *Sāramāyañcu sindūram parayunnen nirākulam /* [24]

I am going to explain the nature of five kinds of *sindūras* for the information of Keralites.

The text is composed in simple Malayalam verses. The text begins with a benedictory verse.

> *Itrailokyamaśeṣavum paṇiyumen brahmāvumaddakṣanum*
>
> *Vṛtrātriyumaśvinītanayarum mukkaṇṇanum kaṇṇanum /*
>
> *ātreyadyarumatrayalla vaṭivil śrī vāhaṭācaryanum*
>
> *śāstrajñan mama vāsudeva guruvum citte vasiccīṭaṇam //* [25]

The creator of the three worlds brahmā, Viṣṇu and Śiva; Kṛṣṇa, Ātreya, Aśvins Vāgbhaṭa, and teacher Vāsudeva are always be with in my mind.

In the next *śloka* the author pays homage to his guru Vāsudeva. In the following verse the procedures to prepare five types of *Sindūras* are mentioned. The author declares that even though there are various methods to prepare *Sindūras*, he accepts the method named *gajapuṭa*.

puṭapākattinanekakramam collunnuṇṭavayil

peṭum gajapuṭam koṇṭulla Veppāṇitil. // [26]

The purification process of five type of *Sindūras*, and the dosage prescribed for various diseases are mentioned. The author also proclaims that the method prescribed in *Sindūramañjarī* is neither his own nor new. This can be inferred from the following verse.

nūnam nūtanamallitente kṛtiyalla vyāja(?)

siddhauṣadham // [27]

In the concluding verse the author warns the physicians that this type of medicines should be prescribed after proper diagnosis of the disease according to other texts.

Sūtrasthānārthasāram suvimalamatiyil sūkṣmamāy saṅgrahiccum

Mātrakālatridoṣasthitiyuṭe nilayum sātmyavum nallavaṇṇam /

Netrattāl kantariññum karamatilamarum pañcasindūraratnam

Sūtram nokki prayogicciṭumalavilavan keli nīlepparakkum. // [28]

The text contains the purification process of medicinal materials like Sulphur, Copper, etc. also in the appendix. It also gives a warning against the use of impure medicinal materials. The impure Sulphur kills the user and the same Sulphur in the pure from cures and gives life to the user; this is depicted as follows:

gandhakam mutalāyulla sādhanaṅṅalkkaśeṣavum

vīryamerum viṣam mūlamennu vaidyaprasammatam /

śuddhiceyyātakattāyāl siddhikūṭumasamśayam

śuddhiceytupayogiccāl siddhikkum rogaśāntiyum // [29]

It is remarkable to note that the author observes that this type of treatment with *Sindūras* and *Bhasmas* are suitable to the new times.

Palajanavumidānīm maṭṭumāttunnamūlam

Cilasamayamitellām nallavaṇṇam phalikkum. [30]

The authors hostile attitude to the allopathic treatment that can be inferred from the *śloka*.

yūropyante viṣam kalarnnoru

marunnentinu montunnu nām. [31]

Why we are interested in taking the poisness medicines of the Europeans ?

The purification process in the Appendix, concludes with the salutation thus:

ātreyanum punaragastyanumatrayalla

Hārītanum carakanum gurunāthanum me /

Colkkoṇṭa vāhaṭasuviśruta suśrutādi

Prācīnavaidyarumenikkavalambamennum. // [32]

I always depend on Ātreya, Agastya, Hārita, Caraka, My teacher, Vāhaṭa, suśruta, and the Vaidyaparamparā (predecessors) before me.

Thus it can be inferred that *Sindūramañjarī* is a text belonging to *Siddha* tradition. It has influenced very much the Keraliya Āyurveda.

Prayogasamuccayam

It was written by Koccuṇṇī Thampurān of Cochin Royal family belonging to the latter half of the 19 AD. The work contains 25 different types of toxins and their treatments. Characteristics of different types of snakes, rats, spider, etc. are described in detail. The treatments evolved out of his own personal experiences and some special preparations are given in the text. The text consists of 11 chapters. The chapters are technically called as *paricchedas*. In the preface to the work Puthezhathu Raman Menon suggests that the work is mentioned by Koccuṇṇi Thampurān as *Prayogasamuccayambhāṣa.*[33] So it seems to be a translation of a Sanskrit text available at that time. He, a friend of Koccunni Thampuran, recollects the memories of Koccunni Thampuran thus; Myself was treated by Koccunni Thampuran several times and he has the ability to predict the future of the patient even from the behavior or the conduct of messegers (*dūta's*). There is a separate chapter allotted for this purpose. The 10th chapter of the work is named as *dūtalakṣa.*

The text begins with the salutation to *Pūrṇatrayīśa*, the family god of the Cochin royal family thus :

sarpādhivāsan hari sarpāridhvajajanaśeṣaguṇanilayan /

tṛppūnitturayappan hṛtpūvil kimapi me vilaṅgiṭeṇam // [34]

Let Hari, reclining on the serpentine conch, taking 'Garuḍa', the divine eagle, as his totem, the abode of all the virtues, the deity at Tripunithura, be within my heart.

In the first *pariccheda* Koccuṇṇi Thampuran declares that he is the son of princess Kāvamma and the nephew of great Koccuṇṇi Thampuran, an adept in toxicology from whom he studied toxicology (Viṣatantra).

kāvammarājñiyuṭe sūnu kṛpārasārdra –

bhāvan viṣamayacikitsaka mauliratnam /

koccuṇṇiyāya mama satguru pūrvajātan

koccuṇṇi bhūpati kaniññu tuṇacciṭeṇam. // [35]

It is interesting to go through a verse while describing the nature of poison among snakes, which throws light on the keen observation of Koccuṇṇi Thampuran thus

vellattil vīṇa pāmbinnu viṣamettam kṣayicciṭum

peṭiccatinnum kākolam nitarāmalpamāyvarum /

krīḍakoṇṭu talarnnuḷḷa pāmpinnum punariṅgine

pāññupāññanyadeśattu cennatinnum kṛśam viṣam /

kīriyoṭettu tottiṭṭu pāñña pāmpatinnum punaḥ

maṇḍūkādikale tinnaneravum svalpamām viṣam /

viṣaśśāntivaruttunnoroauṣadhattinte kīzhile

cirakālam kiṭannoru pāmpinnum viṣamalpamām // [36]

The snakes in the following conditions are of lesser poison.

1)   when it falls in to water.

2)   when it is frightened.

3)   after intercourse

4)   roaming a long distance.

5)   after fighting with mongoose.

6) after taking food.

7) when they live under medicinal materials.

Koccuṇṇl Thampuran did not collect any fees not only for the treatment but also for the medicines. His only aim was the well being of the human society. This can be inferred from the verse given in the 10ᵗʰ *pariccheda* of the text. There he observes thus

Yāgādikarmaṅṅal palatum ceytilum tadā /

viṣārttarakṣaṇattoṭu sāmyamallennu kelppitu. // [37]

Giving life to patient is better than doing thousands of *yagas.*

Moreover one thing that deserves special mention, is that Koccuṇṇi Thampuran was accessible to all human beings irrespective of caste and creed.

Vātarogaciktsā Saṅgraha

It is work by K.Narayanan Vaidyar. This is published in 1935 AD by S.D Reddyar & Sons, V.V press, Kollam. In the introduction the author explains the reason for writing this book. There are so many Āyurvedic books for different subjects, but not so for *vātavyādhi* (rheumatics). In this book he explains thirty six varieties of *vātavikāra* which are not available in authentic Āyurvedic texts.[38] All the specific signs and symptoms with treatments are given. Treatments are mentioned out of his personal practice.

There are also a number of Āyurvedic Malayalam works available in Manuscript Library at Madras; which need separate study. Only those texts, which have direct connection with Sanskrit Āyurvedic sources, and are of wide popularity among present physicians of Kerala are dealt with above.

References

1. *Cikitsāmañjarī*, I –1, p.3

2. *Keraliya Sāhitya Caritram* Vol I, p.512

3. *Ibid.*

4. *Cikitsāmañjarī*, Preface, p.i

5. *Ibid.*, p.35

6. *Ibid* ., p.448

7. *Sarvarogacikitsāratna* I-1

8. *Bṛhadāraṇyakopaniṣad.* -

9. *Ibid* ., p.77

10. *Aṣṭāṅgahṛdaya*, sūtrasthāna, 5/19

11. *Ibid.*, p.316

12. *Aṣṭāṅgahṛdaya*, cikitsāsthāna, 22/74

13. N.V Krishnankutty Varriar, *Āyurveda caritram*, p.349

14. *Ibid* p.131

15. N.V Krishnankutty Varriar, *Āyurveda caritram*, p.350

16. *Sarvarogacikitsānūl*, I-1

17. *Mahāsāram* – M.K Vaidyar (ed.).I.1

18. *Cikitsākacintāmaṇi*, K.G. Paramesvaran Pillai, (ed.) p.28

19. *Agastyavaidyacandrikā.*, Indroduction p.1

20. *Ibid.*, p.31

21. *Ibid.*, p.33

22. *Keraliya Samskṛta Sāhitya Caritram.*, Vol- I . p. 506

23. Vaṭakkumkur, *KSSC* Vol. IV, p.240

24. Narayanan Moos, *Sindūramañjarī* Introduction, p.35

25. *Ibid.*, verse.2

26. *Ibid.*,13

27. *Ibid.*,26

28. *Ibid* ., concluding verse

29. *Ibid.,* appendix verse.4&5

30. *Ibid.,*36

31. *Ibid.,*37

32. *Ibid.,* concluding verse

33. Koccuṇṇi Thampuran, *Prayogasamuccayam*, Preface- IX

34. *Ibid.,* p.1

35. *Ibid.,* p.5

36. *Ibid.,* p.43

37. *Ibid.,* p.44

38. K. Narayana Vaidyar, *Vātarogacikitsā saṅgraha*, p.35.

CONCLUSION

This work has been the investigation into the Kerala Āyurvedic Tradition and its continuation by Keralite authors through their Sanskrit works on Āyurveda against the backdrop of the evolution of Kerala culture. Kerala was a part of a larger kingdom named *Chentamizhnāḍu* which existed from Tirupati to Kanyākumari. Thus the history of Kerala is immersed in the history of Tamil Nadu reflected in the Ancient Tamil works like *Akanānūru, Puranānūru* etc.

To explore out the Kerala tradition of Āyurveda, firstly origin of Āyurveda from Indus Valley and its transition from magico religious (*daivavyapāśraya*) treatment to empiricorational (*yuktivyapāśraya*) treatment as reflected in the authentic texts of Āyurveda, are traced. The legal contempt of physicians for about 1000 years mentioned in the *smṛti* texts (Law books) are described. The role of Buddhist *śramaṇas* in the development of Āyurveda is critically assessed and arrived at a conclusion that actually they were responsible for the development of Āyurveda contrary to the notion that Buddhism arrested the development of Āyurveda.

Basic principles of Āyurveda like *pañcabhūta* theory, *tridoṣa* theory, means of valid knowledge, theory of creation, etc., are dealt with in detail.
Then an attempt is made to trace the evolution of Āyurveda in Kerala and to give an account of some special therapies exclusively developed and practised in Kerala. Due to the non-availability of references to the evolution and culture of Kerala, broad surmises are made on the available materials. For the study of special therapies of Kerala several Āyurvedic healing centers like Kottakkal Āryavaidyaśālā, Nangelil Āyurveda Hospital, Trivandrum Āyurveda College were visited and information about them was collected from the doctors. When I approached traditional physicians who have been practising it, in order to obtain special information about *netracikitsā* for which Kerala has special fame, they told me that they are not ready to reveal the special medicine and that most of the medicines used traditionally by their fore-fathers were already lost. Nowadays

they have been following mainly *Aṣṭāṅgahṛdaya* for *netracikitsā*. For *viṣacikitsā* also the case is the same. They have a list of some special preparations used by their fore-fathers, which they do not want to disclose.

When the Sanskrit Āyurvedic texts by Keralites are examined, it is revealed that most of the texts are some adaptations of *Aṣṭāṅgahṛdaya*. The peculiarity is that some special preparations of their teachers and proved effective by their experience are given at the end of each text. Among the Keralite Sanskrit works, it is revealed that Dh*ārākalpa* is only an independent work by a Keralite, containing different types of *dhārā* treatment. P.S. Varrier's works deserve special mention in this category because they give proper understanding of the modern human anatomy to the traditional Āyurvedic physicians in Sanskrit language. Most of the translations to the technical terms of *Bṛhacchārīra,* etc., were made on the basis of the English terms given in the Appendix by the author himself. But these terms are very much related to Latin roots rather than modern English. For example the translation of the term *bīja* is spermatozoon instead of sperm.

When some widely used Malayalam Āyurvedic works are examined, it is revealed that there are some special preparations which were not mentioned in the primary text like *Carakasaṃhitā, Suśrutasaṃhitā* etc., For example the Āyurvedic Malayalam text *Bālacikitsā* contains references to the preparation and usage of *puliṅkuzhampu*, a special preparation exclusively used by Kerala physicians during post-pregnancy treatments. *Ārogyacintāmaṇi* by Vallathol Nārāyaṇa Menon is a mere translation of *Ārogyakalpaduma* of Kaikkulaṅgara Varrier. Hence, it is not included in this study. Another work which deserves special mention in this category is *Ālattiyūrmaṇipravāḷam*, believed to be a work of Nambi who belonged to *Aṣṭavaidya* clan. The manuscript is available in the Calicut University Manuscripts Library but the deep study of the text is not possible because of the absence of the knowledge of Tamil language. The publication of this work with Malayalam or English translation would be an asset to the field of Kerala Āyurvedic tradition.

An account of some folk medicines widely used by the common mass which came to my attention during my research are given in the Appendix.

Āyurveda in Kerala is a blend of two streams (1) The healing techniques which already existed in Kerala before the advent of Sanskrit Āyurvedic *Saṃhitā* texts. (2) The Āyurveda treatment based on *pañcabhūta* theory and *tridoṣa* theory existed in Sanskrit Āyurveda *samhitas*. The first stream was transmitted orally from generation to generation and some of them appeared in the Āyurvedic works in Malayalam. A large numbers of physicians belonging to the lower strata of society like Vela, Maṇṇān, Ezhava, Kaṇiyān and Kurup (experts in *marmacikitsā*) represent this tradition. The second stream represents the *aṣṭavaidya* tradition that has accepted *Aṣṭāṅgahṛdaya* and other *Samhitā* text as the basis of their treatments. *Sahasrayoga* is another text that deserves special mention accepted by them.

The influence of *Siddha* tradition can also be noticed in the Kerala tradition of Āyurveda.

As far as one can say about the unique therapies of Kerala like *Massage* Therapy and *Dhārā* therapy, etc., are concerned, it may be said that they were the systematisation of knowledge already existed before the advent of Sanskrit *samhitā* texts and later classified under *pañcakarma* Therapy mentioned in *samhitā* texts.

It is hoped that the present survey will prompt Āyurvedic scholars to pursue the subject matter further and establish the link between *Śāstra* and *Prayoga*.

It is high time to collect and codify the rural traditional knowledge among common mass and disseminate that knowledge and methods of preparation of some simple and yet effective medicines to the common mass through *Kuṭumbaśri's,* Educational institutions, etc., This is all-important now to check the undesirable trends of the traditional medicinal knowledge of our fore fathers by the multinational companies and other indigenous companies in the process of Globalisation.

BIBLIOGRAPHY

- Acharya, Jadavaji Trikamji: *Suśrutasamhitā*, Chaukhambha Orientalia,(1980)

- Agarwal R.S.: *Secrets of Indian Medicine*, Sri Aurobindo Ashram, Pondicherry, India, (1983)

- Acharya, Jadavaji Trikamji: *Caraka Samhitā,* Nirnaya Sagar Press, (1941).

- Acharya, Jadavaji Trikamji: *Mādhavanidāna,* Chaukhamba Sanskrit series, (1967)

- Aiyangar Duraiswami (ed): *Tantrasārasaṅgraha,* Chaukhamaba Sanskrit Prathisthan, Delhi, (1992)

- Arber Agness: *Herbal plants and Drugs Their origin and Evolution,* Mangaldeep Publications, Jaipur, (1999)

- Avinash Chandra Kaviratna and Pareshnath Sarma, (ed): *Carakasamhitā,* Kavibhusan, Culcutta, (1925)

- Basham A.L: *The Wonder that was India,* London, (1954)

- Bernal. J.D: *The social Function of science*, London, (1939)

- Bernal. J.D: *Science in History*, Penguin, (1969)

- Bose D.M (ed): *A concise History of Science in India,* New Delhi, (1971)

- Chandran P.V: *Arogyamāsika,* Mathrubhumi publishers, April, (2002)

- Charles Greene Cumston: *History of Medicine*, Gyan Publishing house, New Delhi, (1999)

- Chattopadhyaya, D. P: *Science and Society in Ancient India,* Research India Publication, Culcutta. (1979)

- Chattopadhyaya, D. P: *History of Science and Technology in Ancient India; The Beginnings,* Culcutta, (1986)

- Chidambaran: *Smaraṇikā,* Sree Sankaracharya University of Sanskrit, Kalady. (1999)

- Chopra, R.N. etal: *Glossary of Indian Medicinal plants,* Council of scientific and Industrial Research. New Delhi, (1986)

- Dash, Bhagwan: *A Handbook of Āyurveda*, Concept Publishing company, New Delhi, (1983)

- Dash, Bhagwan: *Massage Therapy in Āyurveda,* Concept publishing Company, New Delhi, (1992)

- Dasgupta. S.N: *History of Indian Philosophy*, 4 Vols, Cambridge, (1922-55)

- David Frawely. Dr.: *Āyurvedic Healing*, Molilal Banarsidas Publishers Pvt Limited, Delhi, (1997)

- Dey. K.L: *Indian Pharmacology A review,* Culcutta, (1874)

- Dominik Wujastyak:, Motilal Banarsidas Publishers. Pvt. Limited, Delhi, Vol I(1998).

- Filliozat. J: *The classical Doctrine of Indian Medicine,* Delhi, (1964)

- F. Max Muller (Tr): *The Upaniṣads*, Dover Publications, Newyork. (1962)

- Ganesh. K.N: *Keralattinte Innelakaḷ*, Kerala Bhāṣā Institute, (1990)

- Ghanckar, Govind: *Abhinavabhārati,* Chaukhamba Samskrta Samsthan, (1968)

- Gupta. B: *Indigenous Medicine in 19th and 20th Century Bengal in C. Laslie, ed; Asian Medicinal systems, A Comparative study,* California, (1977)

- Herman olden berg (ed): *The Vinayapiṭakam*. Mahāvagga. Luzac and company Ltd, London (1964)

- Hoerule. A.F.R: *Studies in the medicine of Ancient India,* London, (1907)

- Iyer, S. Parameswara Uḷḷūr: *Keraḷa Sāhityacaritram,* University of Kerala(1964-65)

- Iyer, Venkitasubrahmania: *Keraḷa Sanskrit Literarture – A Bibliography,* University of Kerala, (1976)

- Iyer, Venkata Subrahmanya(ed): *The Bhelasamhitā* (ed), Central Council for Research in Indian medicine and Homeopathy, New Delhi, (1977)

- John Alexander (ed): *Sarvarogacikitsānūl,* Vidyarambam Publishers, (1996)

- Jones, W.H.S (ed): *Hippocrates*. London (1972)

- Kane. P.V: *History of Dharmaśāstra*, Poona (1930 – 41)

- Keith. A.B: *A History of Sanskrit Literature,* Oxford, (1928)

- Keith. A. B, (Tr): *The Veda of the Black Yajus, School entitled Taittirīya Samhitā,* Motilal Banarssidas, Delhi, (1967)

- Kosambi. D.D: *The Culture and Civilization of Ancient India,* London (1964)

- Krishnan K.V & Pillai Gopala Anakkalil: *Sahasrayoga* with *Sujanapriyā* Commentary, Vidyarambham Publishers, Mullakkal, Alappuzha, (1995)

- Kumar. Anil: *Medicine and the Raj,* Sage Publications, Delhi, (1998)

- Kutumbaih. P: *Ancient Indian Medicine,* Madras (1962)

- Leslie. C (ed): *Asian Medical systems: A Comparative study,* California, (1977)

- Macdonell, A.A: *Vedic Mythology,* Strassburg (1897)

- Maya Tiwari: *Ayurveda secrets of Healing,* Molilal Banarsidas Publishers Private Limited, Delhi, (2003)

- Mehta. P. M, (ed): *Carakasamhita,* Jamnanagar, (1949)

- Menon, A. Sreedhar: *Keraḷa caritram,* National book stall, Kottayam (1967)

- Menon, A. Sreedhar: *A Survey of Kerala history,* S.Visvanathan Pvt Ltd. Sep(1991)

- Menon, V.M. Kutti Krishna: *Aṣṭāṅgahṛdayam, Sūtrasthāna with Malayalam Translation & Commentary,* Department of Cultural Publication, Government of Kerala, (1988)

- Monier Williams. M: *Sanskrit – English Dictionary,* Oxford, (1899)

- Moos, N.S, Vayaskara (ed): *Vaidyamanorama,* Vaidyasarathy Press (Pvt) Ltd. Kottayam, (1979)

- Moos N: *Vaidyaratnam: Medical journal,* Vol -2, Quarterly, Sep-Nov, (2003)

- Moos. N.S.: *Āyurvedic Treatments* of Keraḷa, Vaidyasarathi Press (1983)

- Mukhopadhyaya.G: *History of Indian Medicine,* Culcutta (1922-29)

- Murthy, Srikantha K.R: *Clinical Methods in Āyurveda.* Varanasi, Chaukhamba Orientation, (1983)

- Murthy, Srikantha (ed): *Aṣṭāṅgasaṅgraha,* Krishnadas Academy. (1998)

- Murthy, Srikantha (ed): *Aṣṭāṅgahṛdaya,* Krishnadas Academy, (2000)

- Nambootiri, D. Damodaran (ed): *Cikitsāmañjarī,* Vidyarambam Publishers, Mullakkal Alappuzha, (1999)

- Nambootiri, D. Damodaran (ed): *Yogāmṛtam,* Vidyarambam Publishers, Mullakkal, Alappuzha, (1999)

- Narayanan, M.G.S.: *Kerala Caritrattinte Aṭisthānaśilakaḷ,* Lipi publications, Calicut, July, (2000)

- Needham, J: *Science and Civilization in China,* Cambridge, (1965)

- N.S Sonatakke and C.G Kashikar (ed): *Ṛgveda samhitā* with the Commentary of Sāyaṇācārya Vaidika, Samshodana Maṇḍala Poona, (1933-1951)

- Pāccumūttatu, Vaikkam: *Sukhasādhaka,* Śraddhā Books, Kochi, Sep. (2000)

- Panikkar. K.N: *Culture, Ideology and Hegemony*, Tūlikā Publishers, New Delhi, (1998)

- Paulose, K.G Dr. (ed): *Scientific Heritage of India*, (Āyurveda), Govt. Sanskrit College Committee, Tripunithura, July (1992)

- Paulose.K.G., *Pūrṇatrayī*: Govt. Sanskrit College, Tripunithura, Vol. XXII (1996).

- Paulose, K.G Dr. (ed): *Indian Health Care Tradition A contemporary view,* Department Of Publications, Ārya Vaidyaśāla, Kottakkal, (2003)

- Paulose K.G, Dr. (ed): *Seminar Prabandhaṅṅal,* Department of Publications, Arya Vaidya Sala, Kottakkal, January, (2004)

- Piggot. S: *Prehistoric India*, Penguin Books, (1976)

- Pillai, Gopala Anekkalil (ed): *Ārogyarakṣākalpadruma,* Devi Book stall, Koṭuṅṅallūr June (1993)

- Pillai, K. Paramesvar: *Agastayvaidyacandrika,* Vadayattukotta (ed) Devi Books stall, Koṭuṅṅallūr, February (1998)

- Pillai, Gopāla Ānekkaḷḷil: *Bālacikitsā,* Vidyārambam Publishers, Alappuzha,(1993)

- Pillai, Gopala Ānekkaḷḷil : *Sarvarogacikitsāratna,* Devi Bookstall, Koṭuṅṅallūr, July, (2002)

- Poduvāḷ, Acyuta (ed) : *Bheṣajapaddhati,* Sanskrit college Committee, Tripunithura, (1973)

- Raja, K. Kunjunni Dr.: *The Contribution of Kerala to Sanskrit Literature,* University of Madras, (1950)

- Raja K. Kunjunni Dr.(ed) : *Samskṛta Sāhitya Caritram,* Sāhitya Academy, Trissur, 1986,

- Raja Raja Varma, Vatakkankur: *Keraḷīya Samskṛta Sāhitya   Caritram,* S.S.U.S., Kalady, (1997)

- Ralph T.H. Griffith, (Tr): *The texts of the white Yajurveda,* E.J Lazarus & Co, Banaras, (1957)

- Ralph T.H. Griffith, (Tr): *The Hyms of the Atharvaveda,* The Chaukhamba Sanskrit series office, Varanasi, 1968, Rpt, The Chaukhamaba Sanskrit studies, (1966)

- Ralph T.H. Griffith, (Tr) : *The Hyms of the Rgveda,* Varanasi, The Chaukhamba Sanskrit series office, The Chaukhamba Sanskrit study, V[th] ed., (1971)

- Ravindran, T.K: *Journal of Kerala Studies,* Vol IX, 1982.

- Ray, P.C: *A History of Hindu Chemistry,* Centenary Edition, Shaibya prakasan vibhag, Kolkata, November (2002)

- Richard Garbe (ed): *The Śrautasūtra of Āpastamba,* belonging to the Taittirīya samhitā, with the commentary of Rudradatta, Motilal Banarssidas, (1967)

- Rudolf Hoernle A. F (ed) : *The Bower Manuscript,* Office of the Superintendent of Government printing, India, Archeological survey of India, Calcutta, (1893 –97)

- Sachau. E.C (ed): *Al –Beruni's India.* New Delhi, (1964)

- Sastri, Brahma-Sankara (ed): *Bhāvaprakāśa of Bhāvamiśra* with the *Vidyodini, Hindi Commentary,* Chaukhamba Sanskrit series, Varanasi, (1969)

- Sastri, K.A.N : *Facets in the History of Medicine,* Indian journal of History of Medicine, (1960)

- Sastri, Parasurama (ed) : *Sargadharasamhita,* Nirṇaya Sagar Press, (1962)

- Sastri, Sambasiva (ed) : *Hṛdayapriya,* Trivnadrum Sanskrit Series, (1939)

- Sharma. R.S : *Aspects of political ideas and institutions in Ancient India,* New Delhi, (1959)

- Sharma. R.S : *Material Culture and social formations in Ancient India,* Macmillain, (1983)

- Sharma, Priyamvrat : *Āyurved- Kā-Vaijñānik itihās* (Hindi), Varanasi, (1975)

- Sharma Priyamvrat : *Essentials of Āyurveda*, Motilal Banarsidas Publishers Pvt Limited. Delhi, (1998)

- Sharma, Sankara : *Dhārākalpa*, Vaidyasarathi Press Pvt. Ltd, Kottayam,

- (1956)

- S.N. Sen and B.V. Subbarayappa (ed) : *Śāstram Indiayil* (Tr) by P.T. Bhaskarapanikkar etal Kerala Bhasha Institute, (1996)

- Sree Kumari Amma (ed): *Āyurveda Itihāsam*, Govt. Ayurveda College, TVM, (1986)

- Srisa chandra vasu (ed): *The Aṣṭādhyāyī* of Panini, Motilal Banarsidas, Delhi, (1977)

- Sri. Taradattapanta: *Aṣṭāṅgahṛdaya samhitā* of Vāgbhaṭa, Āyurvedācārya, The Chaukhamba Sanskrit Series Office, Varanasi, (1956)

- Suresh, Dr. : *Physician*: Kerala state Govt. Āyurveda Medical officers-Association, May (2004).

- Takakusu. J: *A Record of Buddhist religion as practiced in India,* London (1966)

- Tampurān, Koccuṇṇi: *Prayogasamuccayam*, Sulabha books, (1999)

- Thapar. R: *A History of India.* Vol I, Penguin (1966)

- Thirumulpad, K. Raghavan: *Āyrvedadarśanam,* Kerala Bhāṣā

- Institute, (1996)

- Thirumulppād, K. Raghavan: *Āyurvedaparicayam*, Nagārjuna

- Publication, (1998)

- Thirumulppād, K. Raghavan: *Aṣṭāṅgadarśanam,* Kerala Bhasa institute, TVM, (1998)

- Thirumulppad, Raghavan Dr, (ed) : *Rasavaiśeṣika,* (Comm)

- Publication wing, Vaidyaratnam Ayurveda College Union, Ollur, July (1993)

- Tripati, Indradev: *Rasaratna samuccaya*, Chaukhamba Samskrta Bhavan, (1997)

- Unithiri, N.V.P Dr, (ed): *Tantrasārsaṅgraha*, with Mantravimarśini commentary Publication division, University of Calicut, November(2002)

- Vaidyar, M. Narayanan: *Carakasamhitā* with Malayalam Commentary Dhanvanthari Printers, Natal, Edakkad, (1993)

- Varghese, Rajan, *Vijñanakairaḷi:* Kerala Bhāṣā Institute, June (2004).

- Varrier, P.V, Dr. (ed): *Ayurvedam Arogyamargam*, Aryavaidyasala, Kottakkal, December (2000)

- Varrier, N.V .Krishnankutty *Āyurvedacaritram,* Āryavaidyaśāla Kottakkal, (1993)

- Varrier, P. K. etal: *Indian Medicinal plants*, a compendium of 500 species, Orient longman, (1994)

- *Varrier.P.S., Dhanvantari*: Ārya Vaidyaśāla, Kottakkal.Vol.12, No.11, 16th August,(1913)

- Varrier, P.S: *Aṣṭāṅgaśārira,* Āryavaidyaśāla, Kottakkal, (1962)

- Varrier, P.S: *Bṛhacchārira*, Āryavaidyaśāla, Kottakkal, Vol 1 and Vol 2 (1969) & (1988)

- Varrier, Raghavan and Gurukkal, Rajan: *Keraḷacaritram,* Vaḷḷathol vidyāpīṭham, Śukapuram(1999)

- Venkata Ramanan. K: *Nāgarjuna's Philosophy*, Harvard, (1966)

- Vishva Bandhy, etal (ed) : *Atharvaveda (Śaunaka) with Padapāṭha and sāyaṇācārya's comentary,* Hosiapur, Vishvesharanand Vedic Research Institute, (1960 –1962)

- V.V. Sivarajan and Indira Balachandran: *Āyurvedic Drugs and their plant source*, Oxford and IBH publishing Co. Pvt Ltd, Delhi(1996)

- William Dwight whitney (Tr) & Charles Rootwell Lanman (ed): *Atharvavedasamhitā,* Motilal Banarasidas, Rpt. Delhi, (1968)

- Winternitz : *A history of Indian Literature,* Calcutta. (1927-33)

- Zimmer. H.R : *Hindu Medicine*, Baltimore (1948)

- Zysk G. Kenneth. : *Medicine in the Veda*, Indian Medical Tradition (ed), Delhi, (1996).

- Zysk G. Kenneth. : *Ascetism and Healing in ancient India,* Motilal Banarsidas, Delhi, (1998)

ILLUSTRATIONS

A. DHĀRA

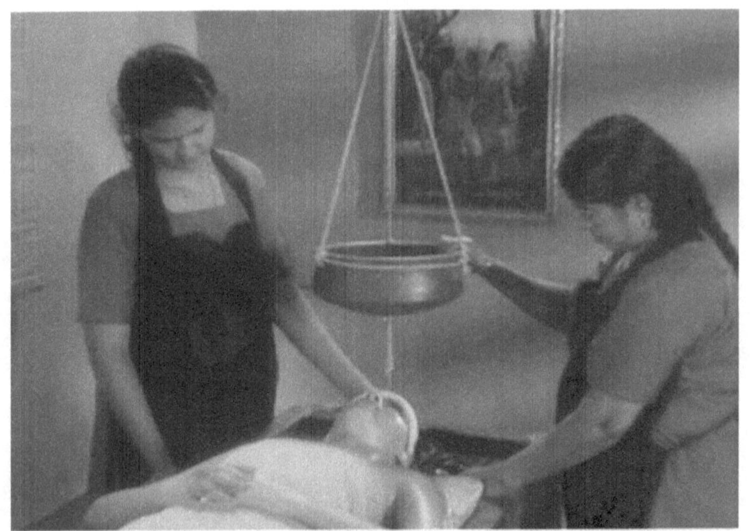

B. ŚIROVASTI

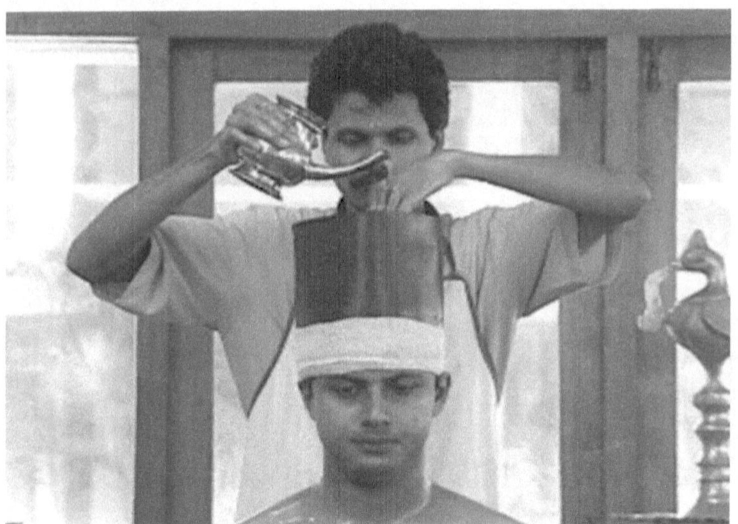

C. UZHICCIL

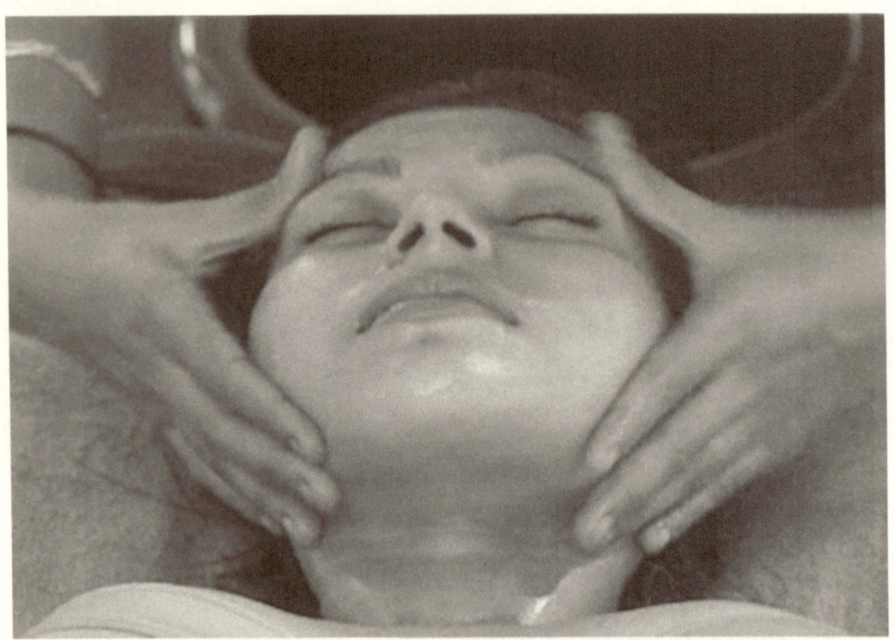

D. NAVARAKKIZHI

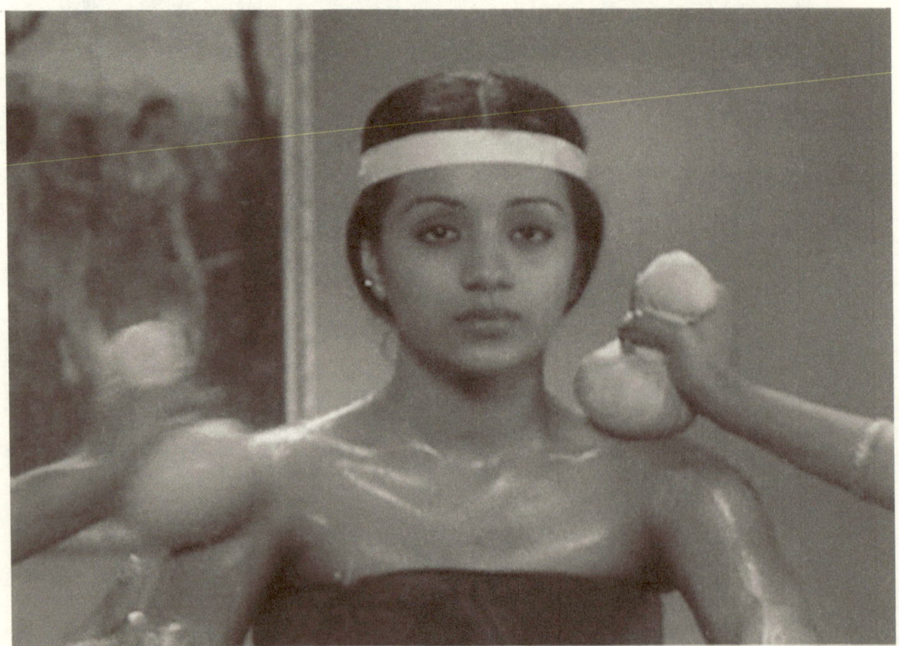

E. POṬIKKIZHI

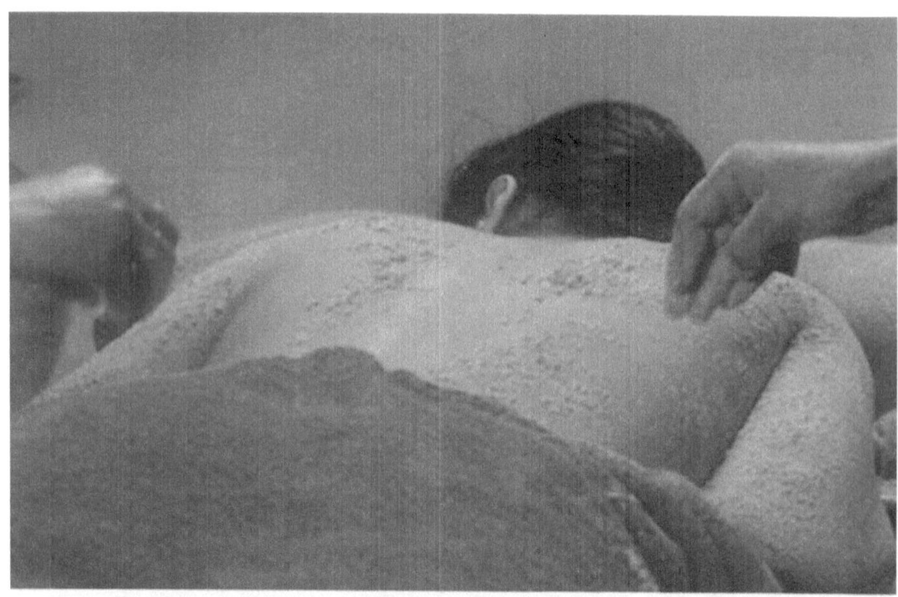

F. NELLIKKĀTTALAM

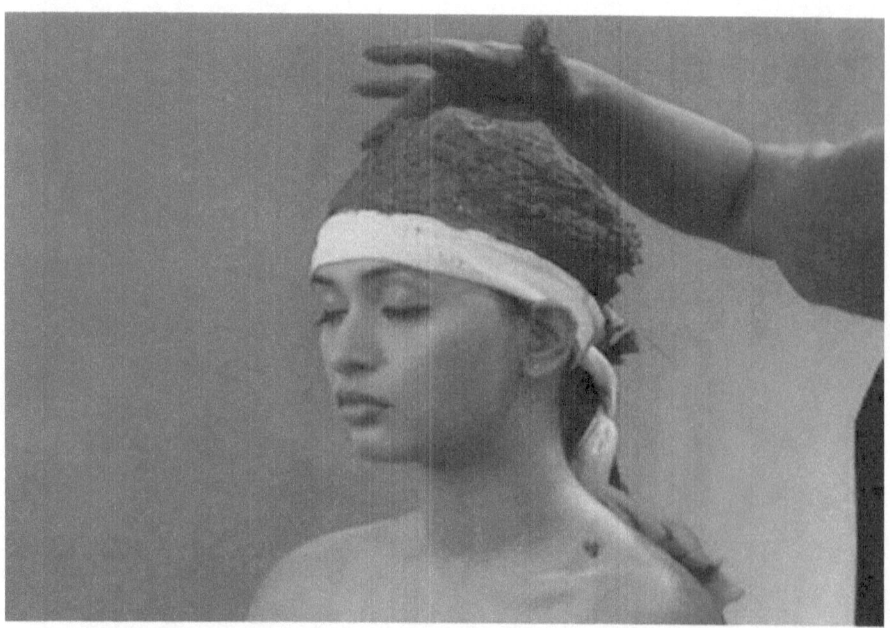

G. UROVASTI

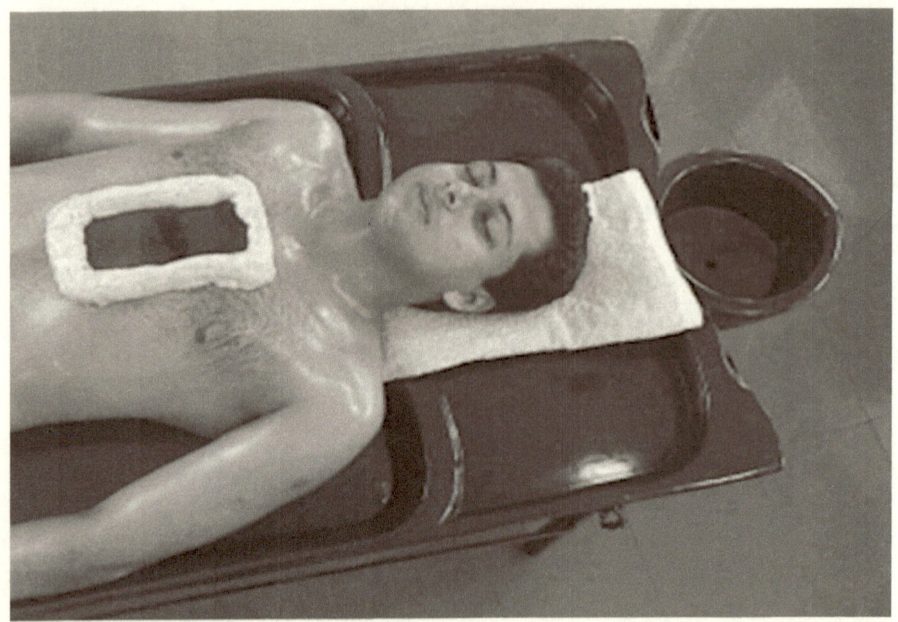

H. PIZHICCIL

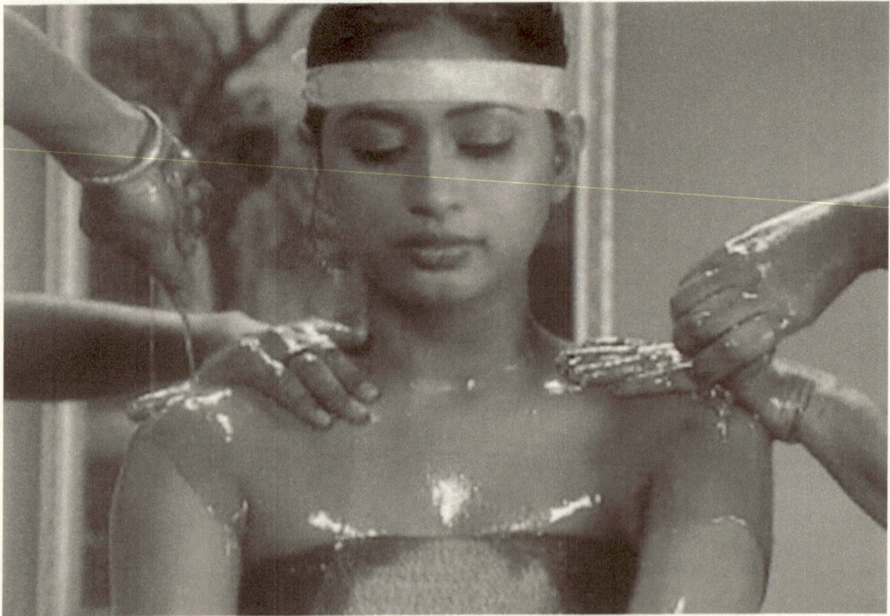

विविध यंत्र शस्त्र

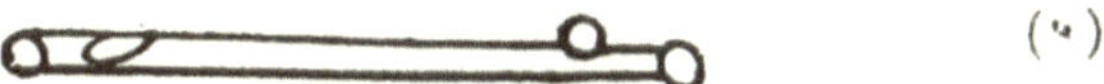

(५)

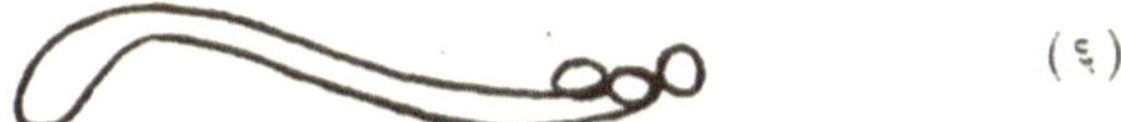

(६)

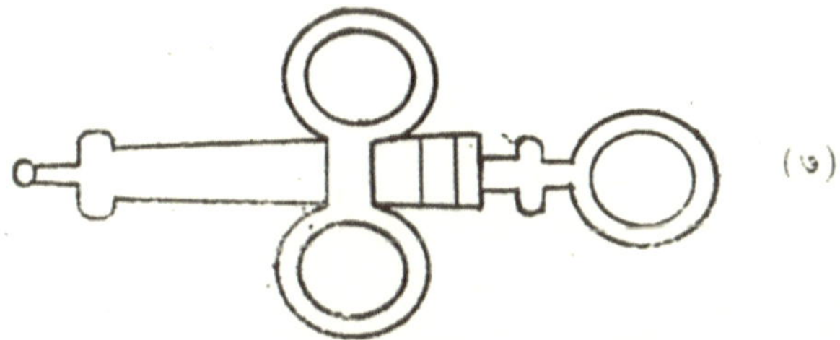

(७)

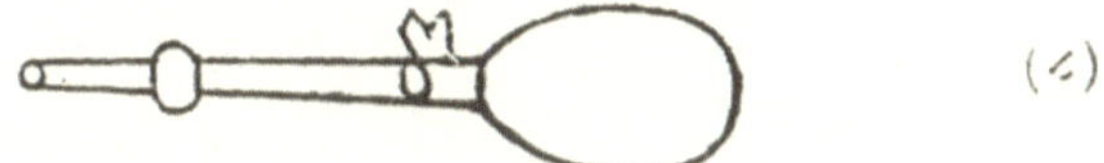

(८)

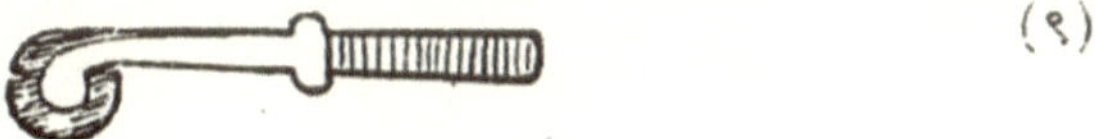

(९)

(१०)

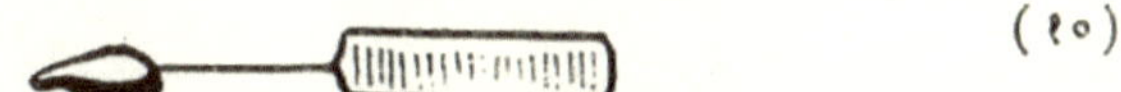

५, ६. फीमेल कॅथेटर   ७. मेटल सिरींज   ८. बस्ति यंत्र
९. कुठारिका शस्त्र   १०. त्रीहिमुख शस्त्र

APPENDIX

LIST OF SOME RURAL MEDICINES

Disease	Medicine
1. Stomach pain	Take the juice of holy basil (*karintuḷasi*) with salt.
2. Night blindness	Grind pepper in curd and use it as an eye ointment.
3. Bronchial troubles especially for *āstama* ('*ekkam*')	Use hair oil prepared out of the following ingredients (1) Take the juice of '*tumba*' (Trichodesma indicium) whole with root (*samūlam*). It should be collected before flowering, 1/4 portion. (2) Juice of a dry coconut, 1/4 portion (3) Gingely oil, 1/4 portion The above juices are boil with 6 '*kazhañj*' of paste of the root of '*tumba*' and filter it in '*manalpāka*' stage and use it after mix with Camphor at the '*patrapāka*' stage.
4. Cuts and bruises	Grind the leaves of '*mūtta kāramullu*' ripened forest pepper in ghee and apply to affected parts. (*murikūṭṭi marunnu*)
5. Fever and cough in children	Boil the leaves of '*panikkūrkka*' (Velliveroides) in a tight bottle and extract the juice and intake it and put in the *neruka* (centre of the head) with or without *rāsnādicūrṇa*

Disease	Medicine
6. Urinary infection	Boil water with *ñeriññil* (land catrops) and take it after cooling.
7. Facial herps and black spots	The juice of the outer covering of ripened arecanut, mix with *eraṭṭimadhuram* (Liquorice) as *kalka* and boil with ghee and use it as facial massage.
8. Hard excrescence on the skin	Take *karuka* (Couch grass), (*pāluṇṇi*) *eraṭṭimadhuram* (licorice) and gingely in equal proportions and roast them in ghee and apply to the affected parts.
9. Scurf (*poḷīla*)	Put the powder of '*ponkāram*' (Borax) in lemon juice and mix it with sandal paste and apply to the affected parts.
10. Corn (*āṇi*)	Add the powder of *ponkāram* in the juice of ripened cyst of arecanut and butter and apply to the affected parts.